Evaluation of the Adolescent Patient

IRIS F. LITT, M.D.
Professor of Pediatrics
Director, Division of Adolescent Medicine
Stanford University School of Medicine
Stanford, California

HANLEY & BELFUS, INC./Philadelphia
MOSBY–YEAR BOOK/St. Louis • Baltimore • Boston • Chicago • London
Philadelphia • Sydney • Toronto

Publisher: HANLEY & BELFUS, INC.
210 S. 13th Street
Philadelphia, PA 19107
(215) 546-7293

North American and worldwide sales and distribution:

MOSBY–YEAR BOOK, INC.
11830 Westline Industrial Drive
St. Louis, MO 63146

In Canada: THE C.V. MOSBY COMPANY, LTD
5240 Finch Avenue East
Unit 1
Scarborough, Ontario M1S 4P2
Canada

EVALUATION OF THE ADOLESCENT PATIENT ISBN 0-932883-98-2

Library of Congress catalog card number 90-81222

Last digit is the print number: 9 8 7 6 5 4 3 2 1

With love to my sons,
Bill and Bob,
who taught me that parenting teenagers can be a joy!

Contents

Preface

This book has been written as a reflection of the real world of medical care in which a patient—in this context, an adolescent—presents with **symptoms** or **signs** rather than **diagnoses.** The reader will judge from its size alone that the book is not intended to be a "Textbook of Adolescent Medicine." Textbooks are typically organized in such a way that the reader has to know the diagnosis in order to find any information. In using this book, one should be guided to a diagnosis based on the information elicited from the adolescent patient. The information required and the ways and means of obtaining it are described in logical sequence in the book in chapters such as "Approach to the Adolescent Patient," "The Medical History," "Growth and Development," "Review of Systems," and "Physical Examination." The final chapters are on special problems of adolescents and detail evaluation of the patient with problems such as chest pain, eating disorders, or drug abuse.

The ultimate goals of this book are:

1. To increase the comfort of health professionals, both in practice and in training, in caring for the adolescent patient.
2. To recognize the differences between the adolescent and the younger or older patient (and among adolescents at different stages in their development) with respect to history-taking, physical examination (including the signs and staging of pubertal development), and differential diagnosis of signs and symptoms.
3. To maximize the opportunity for health education and anticipatory guidance afforded by the infrequent visits of adolescents to health care facilities.

I hope that the reader will find the book to be a friendly companion and easy to use, and will derive more enjoyment from treating adolescent patients as a result of having read it and periodically referring to it.

Iris F. Litt, M.D.

Approach to the Adolescent Patient

HEALTH PROBLEMS OF ADOLESCENTS

Adolescents have generally been considered as a group to be healthy, so it is not surprising that until relatively recently they have received little medical attention. This has resulted in their being largely ignored in epidemiologic studies, reinforcing the image that their medical problems are few. Within the past two decades, however, concerns about the abuse of drugs and the increasing rates of pregnancy have led to greater involvement of the health professions with adolescents, with the end result that a wide range of health issues have surfaced. It is now recognized that a myriad of health problems might be prevented and/or treated if only there were more contact between physicians and adolescent patients. These health problems fall into the following categories:

1. **Consequences of puberty.** A number of disorders are caused by the very process of growth and development that characterizes puberty. Examples include Osgood-Schlatter disease, slipped capital femoral epiphysis, acne, and dysmenorrhea.

2. **Consequences of psychologic development.** The process of experimentation, which is a normal part of adolescent psychosocial development, can have adverse consequences such as pregnancy, sexually-transmitted disease, or drug addiction.

3. **Infections that occur primarily, if not exclusively, during adolescence.** Some infections that were previously prevalent in young children are now responsible for illness in adolescents, including rubella, rubeola, and mumps. Sexually transmitted diseases occur with higher frequency in adolescents because of their disinclination to practice safe sex. Epstein-Barr

virus and toxic shock syndrome occur disproportionately in the adolescent age group.

4. Adult conditions that may be detectable in their asymptomatic phase during adolescence. Examples include hypertension, carcinoma-in-situ of the cervix, and hypercholesterolemia.

5. Survival of children with chronic (and in some instances previously fatal) illnesses into adolescence. Advances in chemotherapy and surgery have made it possible for more children with chronic disorders to live to adulthood. Problems of compliance with vital therapy and issues of family planning and genetic counseling must be addressed in such adolescent patients.

THE ADOLESCENT'S PERCEPTIONS OF HEALTH STATUS AND NEEDS

The teenager's perception of his or her health status may not coincide with that of health professionals and the discordance may be reflected in nonutilization of the limited health care resources that exist for this age group. Self-perceived health status for the adolescent, as for adults, may be influenced by demographic, cultural, and psychological factors as well as physical factors.

In the late 1960s, a study by Brunswick[5] revealed that health concerns of inner city adolescents included not getting enough exercise or sleep, not eating properly, or smoking. To these can be added the concerns of Texan adolescents one decade later: school, drugs, sex, family, getting along with adults, birth control, sexually transmitted disease, pregnancy, and menstrual periods.[49] Other studies report that adolescents may consider themselves to be in poor health if they have acne, headaches, obesity, dental problems, or even bad breath or "smelly" feet. In one study, concerns about school, sports participation, job prospects, relationship with parents, and being attractive to the opposite sex were rated higher than the possibility of getting AIDS among adolescents with hemophilia.[46] On the other hand, worry about AIDS has become rampant among adolescents currently, even among those without risk factors for the disease, in our experience.

A recent British study found that more than 90% of students rated their health to be fair or good, despite their need for medication (three-quarters), absence from school (one-third), feeling depressed and/or drinking alcohol at least once weekly, or having headaches.[34] During adolescence there appears to be a paradox in self-perceived health status, with one extreme represented by those who feel invulnerable to disease and, accordingly, deny any physical symptoms, and the other by those who exaggerate their discomfort and imagine a serious disorder when none exists, often considered hypochondriacs. The latter extreme may be accounted for by the heightened self-awareness or self-consciousness that often occurs at this time in life. Cognitive developmental changes also favor the latter extreme as a variant of introspection. Mechanic,[37] for example, found more physical and psychological symptoms and higher utilization of health services among those adolescents who rate higher in measures of introspectiveness. Within the adolescent age group there may also be stage-dependent variations in health perception. Millstein and Irwin[41] found younger adolescents to be more concrete in their definition of health, which essentially was perceived as the absence of disease. Older teenagers included more nonsomatic and psychosocial themes in their definition of self-health.

THE MEDICAL VISIT

The adolescent patient brings to the medical visit a variety of concerns, biases, and fears that often inhibit the free flow of information between the physician and patient. The health care provider must make a special effort to put the adolescent at ease, to build rapport, and to establish himself or herself in the role of the teenager's health advocate. A number of factors potentially contribute to or interfere with this goal: the patient's and the provider's gender, the agenda of the visit, the presence of others, the clinical setting, and the stage of development of the adolescent.

Gender

It is difficult to generalize about a teenager's preference for a physician of a specific gender. In our experience, females who request a female physician may do so when prompted by their parents, when they are young or immature, or if they have previously had a positive experience with a female physician or, conversely, a physically or emotionally uncomfortable experience with a male physician. In a study of adolescents in the context of prenatal care, we found that Mexican teenagers were more likely to request a female physician than were Mexican-American or Anglo patients, suggesting that there may be cultural influences in this choice as well.[39]

In addition to the characteristics of the patient, the circumstances of the visit may influence gender preference, as in the case of concern about possible sexually transmitted disease or rape. Under these circumstances, the request is generally for a physician of the same sex as the patient. Intuitively, it may appear appropriate to honor such a request when possible. Alternatively, it may be more therapeutic to provide a caring and gentle physician of the opposite sex, in which case it is appropriate to have a chaperone. Traditionally the presence of a chaperone has been considered more essential when the physician is male and the patient female, but if the adolescent patient is in the process of exploring his or her gender role and sexual preference, it may be advisable to have a chaperone present regardless of the physician's gender, in order to avoid any misunderstanding of the physician's motivation for examination. During examination of the breasts of females or external genitalia of males, it is useful to preface the initiation of the procedure by a statement such as: "I am now going to examine your breasts/testes for lumps. Please pay special attention to the way that I am performing the examination so that you may be able to examine your own breasts/testes in the future." The perception of the examination as an act of "touching" is removed from a potentially embarrassing sexual context to an educational one and is thus rendered more acceptable and effective.

Agenda of the Visit

Although the physician may wish to take advantage of the rare medical visit of the adolescent to provide health education, anticipatory guidance, and preventive health care (see below), it is important to give attention first to the patient's agenda, even if it means scheduling a future visit to accomplish these other important items. Our studies show that compliance by adolescent patients with prescribed medication (specifically, oral contraceptive) has been better when the patient came to the physician for the purpose of obtaining contraception than if birth control had been only on the physician's agenda.[32] The challenge is to motivate the patient so that his or her agenda coincides with that of the physician. We have also found that adolescent patients are more satisfied (and therefore more likely to be compliant with whatever prescribed medical regimen) if they, rather than a parent, had made the appointment.[31] Pregnant adolescents are more satisfied with their interaction with their prenatal care provider if the content of the visit emphasizes obstetric issues, such as preparation for labor and delivery, than if the physician's agenda focuses on prohibitions about smoking or using drugs or alcohol (what is often mislabeled "educational"). These important issues must be addressed in a nonjudgmental manner.

If a patient screening questionnaire (see Appendix 1) has been administered prior to the visit with the doctor, it is important that it be reviewed before the patient's departure, even if little time remains. If any items are found that require additional discussion, the patient should be so informed and another visit set up in the near future for the purpose of fuller exploration of the relevant issues. If such an instrument in any way suggests the possibility of depression, this must be pursued immediately, regardless of time constraints (see pp. 164–168).

The Presence of Others

Adolescent patients typically enter the examining room accompanied by a parent or occasionally by a friend. The presence of a friend, family member, or others will surely affect the comfort of the patient and physician and influence their interaction. Younger adolescents may prefer to have their parents with them, whereas older ones often prefer to be unaccompanied. Their reasons for coming to the doctor will of course play a role. The physician's tasks are:

1. Determine whether it was the parents' or the patient's idea to come to the doctor's office.
2. Find out what the agenda of each is, particularly to learn whether these agendas are congruent.
3. Establish his or her role as patient's advocate.
4. Establish immediately (even before exploring the agenda for the visit) that part of the interview will be conducted with the adolescent alone and that confidentiality will be maintained. If the patient indicates concern about being separated from the parent or friend, the physician must be flexible and defer separation until the next visit, after rapport has been established.
5. Determine if the accompanying person is there because of intrusiveness or possessiveness, or because it is the patient's actual wish.
6. Inform the parents that they will have an opportunity to speak with the doctor after the patient is evaluated, privately if they wish.
7. Allow time to interview the friend, if appropriate and with the patient's approval, and if it appears likely that potentially important information may be gained. Compliance may be enhanced if the friend's potential reservations and concerns are addressed. For example, if the friend has questions about side effects of the oral contraceptives that are being prescribed and is not given the opportunity to raise them during the visit and be reassured by you, he or she will likely bring these questions up with your patient afterward. As adolescents are very vulnerable to peer pressure (to say nothing of being frightened by what they may be told), they are at risk for noncompliance under such circumstances.
8. If the patient's boyfriend or girlfriend has not accompanied the patient, it is advisable to invite him or her to the next visit to enlist support. This is most important in the context of provision of contraception, as one of the most frequent reasons for noncompliance is a boyfriend's disapproval or distrust. Involvement of a "significant other" can also be helpful when medication or other regimens are prescribed for a patient with a chronic illness. In that circumstance, it is appropriate to initiate a dialogue with those

people most important to the adolescent patient. When the adolescent's heterosexual relationship is a serious one, issues such as fertility, genetic counseling, and dangers of pregnancy may subsequently surface. This can be facilitated by earlier interactions among the chronically ill adolescent, his or her physician, and future spouse.

The Setting

The setting will influence the content and conduct of the interaction with the adolescent patient. In recognition of the fact that adolescents are often reluctant or poorly motivated to come to a doctor's office, health care providers are increasingly reaching out to them in settings in which they are more available or more receptive. Health care for adolescents may be provided using any of a variety of models:[10]

- Uni-site, Uni-service: Provision of care for a specific condition or purpose at one site. An example is a freestanding family planning clinic.
- Multi-site, Uni-service: As above, but service is provided at more than one site. An example is Planned Parenthood or municipal venereal disease clinics.
- Multi-site, Multi-service: Provision of care for a number of conditions at many sites. An example is a medical school–based adolescent health program with outreach services at community sites (such as a detention facility, secondary school, college health service).
- Uni-site, Multi-service: Provision of health and other services (for example, legal, vocational, educational, recreational) at one site. An excellent example of this model is The Door in New York City.

School-based clinics, long a tradition in many other countries, currently are being developed in many parts of the United States as a way to reach adolescents not receiving necessary health care.[40] Although often targeting sexually active teenagers in need of contraception, such programs generally provide a wider range of health services to this medically underserved age group and, in so doing, avoid potential stigmatization of students seen using them. Student health services at the college level have a much longer history, however. Over the past two decades, ongoing programs for delivery of health care to disenfranchised youth in detention facilities, storefront clinics, and even mobile vans have appeared, as well as in acute care settings such as rock music concerts.

It is apparent that the physician's interaction with the adolescent patient will be influenced by the setting in which it takes place. If the agency providing health care is viewed by the teenager as being adversarial or supervisory, an implicit threat to confidentiality—to say nothing of suspicion of motives of the health care provider—may be perceived, interfering with the development of an appropriate physician-adolescent patient relationship. In such settings, the physician may also be pressured by conflicting allegiances and obligations. As a result, efforts should be made to clarify the limitations, as well as potentialities, of the relationship. This type of situation often restricts health care provision to acute care for specific conditions. It is therefore appropriate that such episodic care be supplemented by creating links with community resources for follow-up.

The Adolescent's Stage of Development

The adolescent's progress in mastering the Tasks of Adolescence (Table 1) will influence not only the content and agenda of the visit but the quality of the physician-patient interaction and subsequent compliance with recommended therapy:

Establishing Independence. This, the earliest of the tasks of adolescence, relates to the need for the teenager to separate emotionally from his or her family. According to studies by Offer,[44] this process is usually accomplished smoothly. When rebellion does occur, it is typically symbolic and restricted to one specific arena such as dress or hair length. Conflict and upheaval associated with the separation process will have reverberations in the teenager's relationship with the physician. Those in conflict with their parents will be less satisfied with their physician and less compliant with prescribed medication, suggesting that feelings toward parents may be generalized to other adult authority figures.

Establishing a Sense of Sexual Adequacy. The teenager trying to integrate recent pubertal development of secondary sex characteristics with newly experienced sexual feelings will be potentially vulnerable in the context of a medical evaluation. This may be manifested by self-consciousness about these changes, with the adolescent imagining that such development is in some way abnormal or feeling guilty about having engaged in masturbation, petting, or intercourse. Any of these concerns may render the adolescent a reluctant patient, believing that the physician is capable, through the process of the physical examination, of discovering everything he or she wishes to keep secret. The patient will therefore be attentive to the physician's facial expressions throughout the examination and quick to attribute significance to a real or imagined frown. "Am I normal?" is the unasked but omnipresent question in the mind of the adolescent, particularly when it comes to sexual development. For example, the male

TABLE 1. Developmental Tasks of Adolescence

Developmental Tasks of Adolescence
Independence (Autonomy)
Sense of Sexual Adequacy
Educational/Vocational Goals
Positive Self-image
Capacity for Intimacy

adolescent with gynecomastia often worries that his large breasts represent a deviation from true "maleness." For another adolescent, normal concerns about sexual adequacy may have been threatened by surgery near or involving reproductive organs, by delay in pubertal development, or by the experience of an unsuccessful attempt at tampon insertion. The teenager grappling with confusion about sexual preference may find an examination even more threatening.

Establishing Vocational and Educational Goals. When vocational plans are at odds with physical realities, the physician may need to intervene and help to redirect the teenager toward a goal that is more consonant with the limitations of projected body habitus or posed by chronic illness.

Developing a Positive Self-image. Adolescence is a critical time for consolidation of self-image, so as to integrate the physical, social, and emotional pressures and changes experienced during this period. Poor self-image contributes to difficulties in the health care setting, as it does in the other arenas of adolescent functioning. Poor self-image is one of the strongest predictors of early adolescent sexual activity and pregnancy, as well as of noncompliance with medications or medical advice.

Developing the Capacity for Intimacy. Adolescents who view their bodies as disfigured or unattractive are unlikely to allow an intimate relationship to develop. Physicians who are sensitive to this possibility will have numerous opportunities to reassure the teenager about his or her normality, as in a male adolescent with gynecomastia, for example. When the physical defect is real, however, the physician may play a role in recommending corrective surgery or appropriate medical intervention. [I am reminded of Laura, a 19-year-old with Crohn disease, who was engaged to be married. When asked if she was in need of contraceptive information, she indicated that she did not plan to have intercourse, as she "was saving herself for marriage." When next seen, however, she admitted that she had broken her engagement because she couldn't face the possibility of her fiancé seeing the perineal fistulas she had developed (which she had not revealed to her physician). A course of steroids and parenteral nutrition were instituted and the fistulas healed.]

Level of Cognitive Development

Most of the information about cognitive processes in adolescence has been based on the work of Piaget (in Flavell[15]), which focused on the development of logic and mathematical operations in relationship to chronologic age. In his organizational scheme, there are four stages of cognitive development: (1) infancy, the stage of sensorimotor functioning; (2) early childhood, the preoperational stage exemplified by egocentric thinking; (3) middle and late childhood, the stage of concrete operational logic; and (4) the last stage, that of formal operational logic reached during adolescence.

Recently, claims for universality of Piaget's structural stages and for generalizability beyond the domains of the mathematical and scientific have been called into question as alternative theories have emerged.

Work by Flavell[15] and Keating[22] has suggested that there is a more linear and gradual change in cognitive development and that differences may exist between individuals that are domain-specific. The focus is now on both the content and the process of cognition, with consideration of the influence of motivation on both. It appears, for example, that the 11–14 year age range is transitional in the process of developing ability to evaluate theoretical evidence. Attempts at correlating changes in cognition with those of pubertal maturation have not been successful, despite earlier curricular decisions based on hypothesized growth spurts in cognitive abilities.[13]

For the physician caring for adolescents, the issue of the patient's ability to process information is relevant to the success of therapy or ability to prevent illness. In deciding when confidentiality should be extended to the adolescent patient, the physician must assess whether the patient is capable of understanding the theoretical, abstract consequences of failure to follow medical advice and to act in a "mature" and "responsible" manner with regard to his or her health. There is, unfortunately, no simple paper-and-pencil test for assessing cognitive maturity, and the physician must exercise judgment in making this decision and be willing to modify the situation in response to the patient's actual behavior.

Summary

The important foci of the physician's approach to the adolescent patient:

Privacy	Advocacy
Confidentiality	Education
Interaction	Reassurance

Medical Evaluation of the Adolescent Patient

TASKS

1. To assess the adolescent's functional status.
2. To identify specific areas of dysfunction.
3. To intervene to return a dysfunctional adolescent to a level of improved function.
4. To prevent future physical or psychological dysfunction.

EDUCATIONAL CONSIDERATIONS

Health habits and practices established during adolescence are likely to determine the health status of the patient and the patient's family, both present and future.

Self-examination of the breasts is one example of a common health practice that is taught to adolescent females. It has not, however, been proved that this teaching will guarantee continuation into the higher risk adult years. In fact, a recent study conducted by Cromer[11] suggests that it may not be continued even for a short period of time. It has been our experience, however, that many girls teach and remind their mothers to perform this practice. Teaching of testicular self-examination does appear to be effective during the adolescent years. Moreover, as indicated above, placing the breast (or testicular) examination in the context of a teaching experience removes sexual implications, and is therefore more conducive to a comfortable interaction between physician and patient. It also provides an opportunity to discuss more immediate concerns about breasts or testes such as asymmetry, delayed development, or pain. Much education can be accomplished during the course of the examination without necessarily adding to the length of the visit. Teenagers, extremely curious about their changing bodies and often somewhat hypochondriacal about various aspects of them, respond positively to any information provided during the examination.

Educational topics appropriate for inclusion in the course of the medical evaluation of the adolescent include:

- Pubertal growth and development (particularly normal variations in timing)
- Sexuality
- Medical consumerism
- Drugs/alcohol
- Automotive and cycle safety
- Self-examination
- Prevention of pregnancy and sexually transmitted disease
- Nutrition
- Coping with peer pressure

SCREENING

As for patients of any age, the decision to perform a screening test for adolescents should be based on a thoughtful risk-benefit analysis. The issues pertinent to such an analysis during adolescence include:

1. Are normative data available for this age group?

2. Is the condition common during adolescence? What is the likely yield?

3. Is there appropriate therapeutic or counseling intervention that will follow discovery of the condition?

4. Is the adolescent patient psychologically prepared to handle the information derived from the test? If not, what needs to be done to prepare him or her?

5. What is the cost (in terms of dollars, discomfort, etc.) of performing the test, and is it justified in terms of the other considerations?

6. When is the best time for the test to be performed?

Table 2 lists the tests that are appropriate for adolescents, based on their stage of development and sex.

TABLE 2. Package of Care
The Well Adolescent Visit

	Females	Males
	Early Adolescence (Tanner 2)	
Screening		
Physical	Hematocrit	—
	Urine culture screen	—
	Tuberculin	—
Psychosocial	Self-image	Self-image
	Depression	Depression
	Peer interaction (including sexuality)	Peer interaction (including sexuality)
	School performance	School performance
	Substance abuse	Substance abuse
Health Promotion	Self-examination of breasts	Self-examination of scrotum
	Nutrition counseling	Nutrition counseling
Prevention	Smoking	Smoking
	Cycle safety	Cycle safety
	Automotive passenger safety	Automotive passenger safety
	Immunization update	Immunization update
Anticipatory Guidance	Developing independence	Developing independence
	Dealing with peer pressure	Dealing with peer pressure
	Confidentiality	Confidentiality
	Variations in growth and development	Variations in growth and development
	Dating	Dating
	Preparation for menarche	—
Physical Examination		
Special attention to:	Blood pressure	Blood pressure
	Height, weight	Height, weight
	Skinfold thickness	Skinfold thickness
	—	Grip strength
	Stage of sexual development	Stage of sexual development
	Scoliosis	—
	Goiter	—
	Acne	Acne
	—	Gynecomastia
	Tibial tubercle	Tibial tubercle
	Gait	Gait
Treatment (anything revealed by the above +)	Acne	Acne
	Dysmenorrhea	—

From Litt IF: Adolescent health care. In Green M, Haggerty RJ (eds): Ambulatory Pediatrics IV. Philadelphia, W.B. Saunders Co., 1989, with permission.

TABLE 2. Package of Care
The Well Adolescent Visit *(Continued)*

	Females	Males
	Mid-Adolescence (Tanner 3–4)	
Screening		
Physical	Vision testing	Vision testing
	Hearing testing	Hearing testing
If sexually active	Pap smear	—
	VDRL	VDRL
	Chlamydia culture	Chlamydia culture
	Gonorrhea culture	Gonorrhea culture
Prevention	Automotive safety	Automotive safety
	STD prevention	STD prevention
	Prevention of pregnancy	Prevention of pregnancy
	Vocational/educational planning	Vocational/educational planning
	Obesity/inactivity	Obesity/inactivity
Physical Examination	Breast masses	Gynecomastia
	—	Testicular tumor
	Vaginal discharge	Urethral discharge
	Pregnancy	—
	Late Adolescence (Tanner 5)	
Screening		
Physical	Genetically transmitted diseases	Genetically transmitted diseases
If sexually active	Pap smear	—
	VDRL	VDRL
	Chlamydia culture	Chlamydia culture
	Gonorrhea culture	Gonorrhea culture
If homosexual or	—	HIV
bisexual	—	HIV
Prevention	Automotive safety	Automotive safety
	STD prevention	STD prevention
	Prevention of pregnancy	Prevention of pregnancy
	Obesity/inactive	Obesity/inactive
Anticipatory Guidance	Planning for marriage	Planning for marriage
	Vocational/educational planning	Vocational/educational planning
	Cults	Cults
	Becoming a health-care consumer	Becoming a health-care consumer
	Leaving home	Leaving home
	Moving into work force/college	Moving into work force/college
	Entering military	Entering military
	Health insurance	Health insurance
Physical Examination	Breast masses	—
	—	Testicular tumor
	Vaginal discharge	Urethral discharge
	Pregnancy	Pregnancy
Treatment	Corrective surgery (after growth complete)	Corrective surgery (after growth complete)

Taking the Adolescent's Medical History

GENERAL GUIDELINES

1. Use open-ended questions.
2. Don't use "teen-talk" unless you do so naturally. Adolescents are quick to label such behavior as "phony" and withdraw.
3. Try to spend some time with the adolescent alone without his or her parent. Questions about sexuality and drug use should be explored in the context of a private interview and not in such a way as to suggest a stereotype.
4. Neonatal, immunization, family, and medical history are best obtained from the parent rather than from the teenager, who usually does not have the necessary information (but enjoys hearing it recited by the parent).
5. Allow time to listen to the adolescent's responses to your questions, regardless of length.
6. Be prepared to rescue the adolescents' self-image if a parent is critical in presenting the history.

POTENTIAL SOURCES FOR THE MEDICAL HISTORY

The patient
The parent
Accompanying friend
The school (with permission)
Other health care providers (with appropriate releases)

METHODS FOR OBTAINING THE MEDICAL HISTORY

Questionnaires

Questionnaires have the advantage of providing a large amount of uniformly collected data about the teenager with a minimum of time spent by the physician and are, therefore, cost effective. They provide a useful and productive activity to occupy the patient while waiting for the physician. If they cover areas of psychosocial functioning, they also prepare the patient for the fact that the physician is interested in a broader spectrum than "traditional" physical health issues, and thus may facilitate communications about these matters. Having the patient's responses in hand at the outset of the office visit provides the basis for initiating a more comfortable interaction.

The limitations of questionnaires derive from their impersonality, their resemblance in format to school "tests," the tendency of parents, if present, to attempt to influence or monitor responses, and the difficulty they present for teenagers with reading problems.

Examples

General adolescent health screening (Table 2)
Specific
- Self-concept (Piers-Harris, Appendix 2)
- Autonomy (Appendix 3)
- Compliance (Checklist, Appendix 4)
- Eating Disorders (EDI, Appendix 5)
- Depression Inventory (Beck, Appendix 6)

Interviews

Unless the physician has a prior relationship with the adolescent, it is often difficult to establish immediate free communication. Even if communication was easy with the same patient when he or she was a child, the advent of adolescence may result in some normal guarding and distancing on the part of the teenager, as well as the physician's discomfort. Communication may be facilitated by utilizing "open-ended" questions. Open-ended questions are those that ask about thoughts and feelings. They are preferable to close-ended question because they involve the patient in the interview process and stimulate longer answers. Open-ended questions typically begin with "what," "why," "how," or "could," in contrast to close-ended questions, which characteristically begin with "is," "are," "did," or "do."

Examples

Close-ended Question	Typical Adolescent Response
Do you like school?	Yes/no
Do you get along with your father?	Yes/no

Open-ended Question	Typical Adolescent Response
What do you like best about school this year?	"My English teacher because she treats me like an adult and doesn't hassle me . . ."
What would you like to change in your relationship with your father?	"I would like to get him to stop putting me down all the time. He embarrasses me in front of . . ."

The interview should first address the adolescent's concerns and reasons for seeking medical consultation and define the boundaries of the physician-patient relationship. In such a relationship, the physician will provide confidentiality, except when the information gathered has implications for the well-being of the patient or others (e.g., imminent runaway or suicide). The adolescent patient must in turn demonstrate responsible health behavior. Only after the teenager's agenda is considered should the physician proceed with his or her agenda (e.g., functional assessment, education, etc.).

Projective Tests

A number of studies have examined Rorschach tests in adolescents at different stages of development. Although the results have been somewhat inconsistent, there is general agreement that adolescent boys tend to be withdrawn and inner-directed, whereas adolescent females appear to be stressed by emerging feminity. In the otherwise well-functioning adolescent, these tests do not provide clinically useful information and have no place in routine screening. The Draw-a-Person test, by contrast, has been a useful tool in the hands of clinicians and researchers.[57] The teenager who may be reluctant to expose his or her own feelings may be willing to do so in the second person, that is, by telling a story about the figure he or she has drawn. Accordingly, use of this technique may facilitate communication and suggest areas of concern less accessible by direct interviewing alone.

Observation

Much can be learned by observing the adolescent's appearance (such as dress, as a function of experimentation with various roles; or grooming, as a statement of self-image, affect, or mood, etc.), demeanor and interaction with the accompanying parent.

CONTENT OF THE ADOLESCENT'S MEDICAL HISTORY

Immunization History

A frequently neglected component of the evaluation of the adolescent patient is immunization status (see Table 3 for schedule of immunizations during adolescence). Adolescence is a crucial time in the development of susceptibility to infectious diseases. It is a time when immunity conferred by immunizations during the infancy may be waning; when exposure to certain infectious diseases may result in protection against subsequent disease; and when rapid growth may increase susceptibility to activation of latent infection (such as tuberculosis); and it is the time just before child-bearing, for most.

Td. The last booster of tetanus and diphtheria (Td) is likely to have been administered at the time of entry into school. The first 10-year booster is due in mid-adolescence, at about 15 years of age.

Mumps. Male adolescents who have not had mumps or who have not been immunized against mumps should be immunized to prevent the possibility of painful orchitis and resulting sterility should natural infection occur at this time in life. The possibility for gonadal involvement also exists in females. In those previously immunized, immunity has been documented to persist for at least 17 years and is thought to be life-long. However, recent outbreaks of mumps in older adolescents may prompt reevaluation of this belief.

TABLE 3. Immunization Schedule for Adolescents

Rubella
- Check titer (or store for 3 months and check only if patient becomes pregnant).
- Give MMR booster at 11–12 years of age.

Rubeola
- Give MMR to anyone with uncertain immunization status (especially if immunized prior to 1967 or prior to first birthday).
- Give MMR booster at 11–12 years of age.

Td
- Give at age 14–16.
- Repeat every 10 years.

Mumps
- Administer to postpubertal males who have not been immunized or had physician-documented diagnosis of infection.
- Give MMR booster at 11–12 years of age.

Hepatitis B
- Administer to male homosexuals
- Administer to parenteral drug abusers

Modified from Report of the Committee on Infectious Diseases, American Academy of Pediatrics, 1988.

Rubella. Although it is now routine to immunize at 15 months of age, this was not the practice when many of the current cohort of older adolescents were infants. It is estimated that as many as 20% of adolescent females do not have measurable antibody titers to rubella at the time they are entering their childbearing years. Even among those who have had documented immunization at age-appropriate times, evidence of protective antibody levels may be lacking.[54] Although it is possible that such patients will show an anamnestic response should they have contact with the virus, it is wise to re-immunize those without measurable titers. The current recommendation of the American Academy of Pediatrics includes an MMR booster at 11–12 years of age. Despite the fact that the risk of teratogenic infection in the fetus of a woman who receives rubella immunization is extremely low, it is advisable that precautions be taken to ensure that the adolescent is not pregnant at the time of immunization (perform a pregnancy test) or within the 3 months thereafter (the period of viremia following administration of this live virus) by prescription of contraception.

Rubeola. As with rubella, the age cohort presently at greatest risk for rubeola is the adolescent. Nearly 75% of cases of rubeola currently occur in adolescents and young adults mostly on college campuses and in military barracks. Serious complications of rubeola that are more common in the adolescent include liver disease, pneumonia, and encephalitis. The most recent recommendation of the American Academy of Pediatrics includes a booster MMR at 11–12 years of age.

Tuberculosis. Although it is not recommended in the United States that adolescents receive bacille Calmette-Guérin (BCG) vaccine, it is appropriate that skin tests for tuberculosis be administered yearly. Any adolescent with a positive purified protein derivative (PPD) of tuberculin who has not previously received a year's course of isoniazid therapy should be so treated to avoid the risk of activation of disease during the pubertal growth spurt. Once isoniazid therapy is completed, the patient may be managed as an adult (i.e., treat only if a recent converter or if evidence of active disease).

Hepatitis B. It is recommended that male homosexuals and parenteral drug abusers receive hepatitis B vaccine (American Academy of Pediatrics, 1988).

The other infectious diseases to which adolescents are particularly susceptible, such as sexually transmitted diseases, Epstein-Barr virus infections, and toxic shock syndrome, are not, unfortunately, preventable by immunizations. Other strategies, such as education about vulnerability and methods of risk reduction, are appropriate and timely during the medical visit with the adolescent patient. The psychology of the adolescent is such, however, that feelings of invulnerability and lack of ability to think abstractly often present barriers to the educational approach to risk reduction.

PSYCHOSOCIAL HISTORY

Assessment of the teenager's present and past functioning should be a routine part of the evaluation. Questionnaires, projective tests, interview, and observation will assist in this task. The major focus should be on the adolescent's adjustment within the three major arenas of the adolescent's life: family, school, and peer group.

Family History

Despite the fact that youngsters increasingly turn to peers for counsel during adolescence, the family remains an important influence throughout this period of time. Accordingly, it is helpful for the health professional to inquire about the composition of the family/household, living arrangements, and family interactions and problem-solving styles as part of the evaluation of the adolescent. Steinberg[61] has studied how the adolescent's pubertal development affects family homeostasis. He has found that the advent of puberty has a marked effect on family interaction that is tempered by its timing and the sex of the adolescent. For example, in families in which there is a late-maturing son, the decision-making hierarchy consists of father>mother>son, whereas in the early-maturing adolescent male's family, it is more likely to be father>son>mother. At the apex of pubertal growth, adolescents of both sexes interrupt family conversation more and explain themselves less. Menarche appears to be the pivotal event in Hill's studies,[20] in that it is followed by a 6-month period of disruption characterized by decreased warmth of the mother and increased conflict between parents. It is only in families of early-maturing females (those whose menarche occurred before or during the fifth grade) that this disruption persists. In studies by Brooks-Gunn,[5] on the other hand, appearance of breasts is the crucial pubertal event for girls in terms of effect on family homeostasis.

Assessment of family interaction is facilitated by asking an open-ended question such as: "What would you like to change in your relationship with your father/mother?" Sensitive issues such as alcoholism and incest have been uncovered in response to this question, in our experience. By inquiring, in addition, if there is anything the teenager might wish to change in his or her parents' relationship, issues of marital discord may surface. Marital discord is a frequent cause of depression in teenagers. Depression in teenagers is also often linked to concern about the health of a family member. It is therefore useful to inquire about the family medical history. A family history of suicide, affective disorders, obesity, or eating disorders are important clues to the potential for later development of these or related problems in the adolescent. The presence of a disabled or chronically ill sibling is obviously important in understanding the adolescent's intrafamilial experience and stress. The family's health beliefs, based on cultural background or previous experience with illness, may be important in determining the adolescent's compliance with medication or a therapeutic regimen.

School Functioning

A screening assessment of school functioning should include information about the number of absences and academic achievement in the current school year in relationship to past years. Merely determining the number of days missed or current grades is inadequate for demonstrating a pattern. An increase in absences or decrement in school performance, for example, should signal the need for further inquiry, as either may be a clue to depression or development of school avoidance, regardless of absolute grades or number of days absent.

Peer Group Functioning

Peer group functioning is established by inquiring if the youngster has one good friend with whom he or she can discuss "anything at all." The teenager without such an actual or potential confidant is believed to be at risk for social isolation and resulting depression. Inquiry as to the teenager's position in the developmental sequence of social interactions, described by Chess et al.,[9] assists in assessment of social functioning. These researchers (Table 4) describe a hierarchy of adolescent relationships progressing from: same-sex group dating to mixed-sex group dating, to pairing off with a member of the opposite sex. Within that context, there is typical progression of heterosexual relationships (Table 5), according to the studies of Schofield[58] in England and Sorensen[60] in the U.S. Placing the teenager within this hierarchy will facilitate discussions about feelings of unpopularity, pressures to become sexually active, the need for contraception, and family conflicts

TABLE 4. Hierarchy of Social Relationships among Adolescents

Same-sex groups
Both-sex groups
Dating
Desire for steady dating
Steady dating
Sexual intercourse

Modified from Chess S, Thomas A, Cameron M: Sexual attitudes and behavior patterns in a middle-class adolescent population. Am J Orthopsychiatry 46:689–701, 1976.

TABLE 5. Progression of Heterosexual Relationships

Stage 1:	Dating without physical contact
Stage 2:	Kissing with touching of clothed breasts
Stage 3:	Touching of unclothed breasts or genital apposition
Stage 4:	Sexual intercourse with a single partner
Stage 5:	Intercourse with more than one partner

Data from the studies of Schofield.[58]

about dating. Concerns about homosexual feelings or behaviors may also be discovered by this approach (see below). Inquiry about possible body-image concerns is important in detecting poor self-esteem or the risk for developing an eating disorder. This may be accomplished by administration of standardized tests of self-image (see p. 185) and/or by asking questions such as: "If you could, what would you most like to change about yourself?" and "What do you consider to be your best and worst features?"

THE SEXUAL HISTORY

A sexual history is a necessary part of every adolescent's medical evaluation because it provides vital information about values, concerns, potential contraindications for medications and diagnostic tests, as well as risk factors for sexually transmitted diseases and pregnancy. It is as necessary for the teenager who has engaged in sexual intercourse as it is for the one who has not. Accordingly, it cannot be undertaken solely in response to the health professional's subjective impression of whether or not the adolescent is sexually active.

Developing a sense of sexual adequacy is a developmental task of adolescence. This occurs in response to the timing and influence of puberty, to reactions of peer and family, and to the adolescent's general self-image. Thus, every adolescent has a "sex life" and the physician cannot be selective or avoidant. The sexual history should not be embarrassing to either the patient or health care provider. A mutually productive interaction is facilitiated by discussing sexuality in the parents' absence, and is also a statement of respect for the teenager's desire to protect his or her parents from that which may be upsetting or from that which he or she may wish to keep private. Just as teenagers often feel protective toward parents, they may also feel this way about their physician. Similarly, physicians may feel parental toward youngsters they have known since birth and may have difficulty initiating the necessary inquiry about sex.

There is no right or wrong way to initiate the sexual history. The best approach is one that feels comfortable, and may fall into one of the following categories: the physical development approach, the preventive approach, the social development approach, or the medical approach.

The Physical Development Approach

In the context of obtaining a history of the chronology and pattern of development of secondary sex characteristics, the physician may comment that these physical changes are commonly accompanied by new and often overwhelming emotions that are sexual in nature. In order to ease the transition to discussion of these issues, the physician might address the variety of ways in which "other" teenagers have dealt with the advent of such feelings (for example, masturbation, petting, and intercourse).

The Preventive Approach

In the context of the physician's accepted role in the primary prevention of morbidity, prevention of sexually transmitted disease (STD) and pregnancy as complications of early sexual experimentation may be comfortably discussed in the course of the adolescent's office visit. Without the need for confrontation as to whether such risks are relevant to the patient, the physician may simply state that information about prevention of and testing for STDs and pregnancy is available for any teenager who might benefit from it and that such requests will be kept confidential.

The Social Development Approach

Inquiry into typical weekend activities will help to place the teenager in the hierarchy of social relationships (see Table 4) and, in that way, lead to identification of the patient who is dating. Follow-up with an open-ended question, such as: "Is there anything about your relationship with (the partner's name) that you would wish to change?", is often answered in terms of sexual pressures and conflicts.

The Medical Approach

Because of potential drug interactions with oral contraceptives (Table 6) and their effects on laboratory test results (Table 7), and because certain drugs, immunizations with live viruses, or diagnostic techniques such as x-ray are contraindicated during pregnancy, it is necessary to have accurate information about use of oral contraceptives or the possibility of pregnancy. The physician may feel comfortable stating this as the reason for taking a sexual history.

A sexual history will help to identify adolescents who need contraception or are pregnant, as well as those who are concerned about sexual development or identity, or are at risk for STDs or pregnancy. It also allows concerns to surface about relationships, homosexual feelings, guilt about certain thoughts or behaviors, perceived inadequacies in development of

TABLE 6. Interactions of Contraceptives with Other Drugs

Interacting Drugs	Adverse Effects (Probable Mechanism)	Comments and Recommendations
Contraceptives, oral, with:		
Acetaminophen	Possible decreased analgesic effect (increased metabolism)	Monitor analgesia
	Possible ethinyl estradiol toxicity (decreased metabolism)	Clinical significance not established
Alcohol	Possible increased alcohol effect (decreased metabolism)	Caution patients
Anticoagulants, oral	Decreased anticoagulant effect (increased factor VII and X; prothrombin may decrease)	Use alternative contraceptive
Antidepressants, tricyclic	Possible antidepressant toxicity (decreased metabolism)	Demonstrated in women taking low-dose estrogen contraceptives given imipramine; monitor imipramine concentration
Barbiturates	Decreased contraceptive effect (increased metabolism)	Avoid concurrent use; use alternative contraceptive in epileptics
Benzodiazepines	Possible chlordiazepoxide or IV diazepam toxicity (mechanism not established)	Use with caution
	Variable psychomotor impairment with single doses of oral diazepam and possibly other benzodiazepines (mechanism not established)	Greatest impairment during menstrual pause in oral contraceptive dosage; possibly not with multiple doses of diazepam since tolerance develops rapidly
	Decreased oral oxazepam, temazepam, or lorazepam effects (possibly increased metabolism)	Increased lorazepam or oxazepam dosage may be required
	Possible triazolam or alprazolam toxicity (decreased metabolism)	Based on studies in healthy subjects; clinical significance not established
Beta-adrenergic blockers	Increased metoprolol and possibly propranolol effect (decreased metabolism)	Monitor cardiovascular status
Caffeine	Possible caffeine toxicity (decreased metabolism)	Possibly significant with large doses of caffeine, especially with prolonged use

Continued

TABLE 6. Interactions of Contraceptives with Other Drugs *(Continued)*

Interacting Drugs	Adverse Effects (Probable Mechanism)	Comments and Recommendations
Contraceptives, oral, with:		
Carbamazepine	Possible decreased contraceptive effect (increased metabolism)	Use alternative contraceptive
Clofibrate	Possible decreased clofibrate effect (increased metabolism)	Monitor blood lipids or chlorphenoxyisobutyric acid concentration
Corticosteroid	Possible increased corticosteroid toxicity (mechanism not established)	Clinical significance not established
Cyclosporine	Hepatotoxicity (mechanism not established)	Single case report
Griseofulvin	Decreased contraceptive effect (increased metabolism)	Use alternative contraceptive
Guanethidine	Decreased guanethidine effect (mechanism not established)	Avoid concurrent use
Hypoglycemics, sulfonylurea	Possible decreased hypoglycemic effect (mechanism not established)	Monitor blood glucose
Methyldopa	Decreased antihypertensive effect (mechanism not established)	Avoid concurrent use
Penicillins	Decreased contraceptive effect with ampicillin or oxacillin (decreased enterohepatic circulation of estrogen)	Low but unpredictable incidence; use alternative contraceptive
Phenytoin	Decreased contraceptive effect (increased metabolism)	Use alternative contraceptive
	Possible phenytoin toxicity (possibly decreased metabolism)	Monitor phenytoin concentration
Primidone	Decreased contraceptive effect (increased metabolism)	Use alternative contraceptive
Rifampin	Decreased contraceptive effect (increased metabolism)	Use alternative contraceptive
Tetracyclines	Decreased contraceptive effect (possibly decreased enterohepatic circulation of estrogen)	Use alternative contraceptive

Continued

TABLE 6. Interactions of Contraceptives with Other Drugs *(Continued)*

Interacting Drugs	Adverse Effects (Probable Mechanism)	Comments and Recommendations
Contraceptives, oral, with:		
Theophyllines	Possible theophylline toxicity (decreased metabolism)	Monitor theophylline concentration; opposing effects of contraceptives and smoking, which increases metabolism, tend to offset each other
Troleandomycin	Jaundice (additive)	Avoid concurrent use
Vitamin C	Increased serum concentration and possible increased adverse effects of estrogens with 1 gram/day of vitamin C (decreased metabolism)	Decrease vitamin C to 100 mg/day

From The Medical Letter Handbook of Adverse Drug Reactions, 1989, p 52, with permission.

secondary sex characteristics, or reluctance to touch one's genitalia. These concerns exist for many teenagers, sexually active or not.

While cognizant of the need to provide privacy and confidentiality to the adolescent, the physician must also make provision for the parents to express their concerns and, in turn, to receive anticipatory guidance without breaching the agreement with the patient. Parents in this society vary tremendously in their reaction to their offspring's adolescence and its implications for emerging sexuality and other risk-taking behaviors. These reactions are often related to their own adolescent experience, past experience with the adolescence of their older children, their perception of this child's vulnerability and, in some cases, to their own mid-life career and marital adjustment. Encouraging parents to express concerns and ask questions will often remove barriers to parent-teenager communication. Discussion about sexuality with parents also provides information about the adolescent's concerns that the adolescent might otherwise be reluctant to raise with the physician.

Because of the implications of physical maturity for adult sexual activity in our society, parents may regard pubertal development in their daughters with concern. Without the opportunity to articulate these concerns, they may resort to imposition of stringent curfews, chaperone arrangements, and other behaviors likely to be interpreted by the teenager as expressions of mistrust, and reacted to by rebellion that often includes sexual acting-out, more to test injunctions of control than out of desire for the sexual experience itself. Another common paternal reaction to a daughter's pubertal development is a distancing and cessation of previous physical expressions of affection. Fathers need assistance in this aspect of transition from childhood

TABLE 7. Effects of Oral Contraceptives on Laboratory Tests

Laboratory Test	Effects	Probable Mechanism
Serum, Plasma, Blood		
Albumin	Slightly decreased	Decreased hepatic synthesis
Aldosterone	Increased	Activates renin-angiotensin system
Amylase	Slightly increased (common)	Not established
	Markedly increased (rare)	Pancreatitis
Antinuclear antibodies	Become detectable	Not established
Bilirubin	Increased (rare)	Reduced secretion into bile
Ceruloplasmin	Increased	Increased hepatic synthesis
Cholinesterase	Decreased	Decreased hepatic synthesis
Coagulation factors	Increased II, VII, IX, X	Increased synthesis
Cortisol	Increased	Increased cortisol-binding globulin
Fibrinogen	Increased	Increased hepatic synthesis
Folate	Decreased or no change	Decreased folate absorption
Glucose tolerance tests	Small decrease in tolerance	Several mechanisms proposed
gamma-Glutamyl transpeptidase	Increased	Altered secretion in bile
Haptoglobin	Decreased	Decreased hepatic synthesis
HDL cholesterol	Increased with estrogens and decreased with progestins	Not established
Iron-binding capacity	Increased	Increased transferrin levels
Magnesium	Decreased or no change	Decreased bone resorption
Phosphatase, alkaline	Increased (rare)	Altered secretion in bile
Plasminogen	Increased	Increased hepatic synthesis
Platelets	Slightly increased	Not established
Prolactin	Increased	Not established
Renin activity	Increased	Increased synthesis of renin substrate
Thyroxine (total)	Increased	Increased thyroxine binding globulin
Transaminases	Slightly increased	Not established
Transferrin	Increased	Increased hepatic synthesis
Triglycerides	Increased	Increased synthesis
Triiodothyronine resin uptake	Decreased	Increased thyroxine binding globulin
Vitamin A	Increased	Increased retinol-binding protein

TABLE 7. Effects of Oral Contraceptives on Laboratory Tests *(Continued)*

Laboratory Test	Effects	Probable Mechanism
Vitamin B12	Decreased	Not established
Zinc	Decreased	Shift of zinc into erythrocytes
Urine		
delta-Aminolevulinic acid	Increased	Increased hepatic synthesis
Ascorbic acid	Decreased or no change	Not established
Bacteria	Increased incidence of bacteriuria	Not established
Calcium	Decreased	Decreased bone resorption
Cortisol (free)	Unchanged	—
Porphyrins	Increased (may precipitate porphyrin in susceptible patients)	Increased delta-aminolevulinic acid synthetase
17-OHCS	Slightly decreased or no change	Increased binding proteins
17-KS	Slightly decreased or no change	Increased binding proteins

From The Medical Letter, 21:1979, with permission.

to adolescent relationships, so as to avoid misunderstandings and to build a mature father-daughter relationship that will be comfortable for all. As discussed above, the major familial impact of pubertal development for sons is in their relationship to their mother.

NUTRITIONAL HISTORY

Analyses of adolescents' diets indicate strong food likes and dislikes. Adolescence is a time when restrictive diets may begin as a result of newly espoused religious or spiritual beliefs or simply out of a desire to lose weight. In our study, for example, 61% of adolescent females were found to have engaged in dieting for the purpose of weight reduction. There was a 45% life-time prevalence of use of diet pills in dieting. Also of great concern is the fact that eating disorders typically begin during adolescence (see pp. 129–141). Evaluation of the adolescent includes careful inquiry into both the content and setting of meals.

Iron Deficiency

Among adolescents' least favorite foods are spinach and liver, so it is not surprising that iron deficiency is common in this age group. Development of muscle tissue during puberty also demands increased iron intake in males (18 mg each day). Iron is ordinarily lost in menstrual fluid and in sweat, with both accounting for losses of 0.5 mg daily, with the resulting requirement during puberty of 18 mg daily of elemental iron for females as well. Certain activities, such as running, result in loss of small amounts of blood in the stool. The frequent use of nonsteroidal anti-inflamatory drugs by athletes may be another cause of blood loss in the stool. Iron deficiency has recently been demonstrated in competitive swimmers. Adolescents who engage in strenuous athletic activities have been found to be at increased risk for iron deficiency as the playing season progresses.[56] Because of these findings, as well as the losses caused by sweating, adolescent athletes are at increased risk for iron deficiency. Even before this deficiency becomes manifested in a low hematocrit or hemoglobin, it can be detected in the serum ferritin level.

Motivation for compliance with iron supplementation is not difficult to achieve once the athletes learn that performance is linked to hemoglobin levels and increases as the oxygen-carrying capacity of the blood increases. It is recommended that adolescents be checked for iron deficiency before, during, and after the playing season.

Calcium Deficiency

Another mineral that may be low in the adolescent female is calcium. Because the daily requirement of 2 gm during puberty requires an intake of between 4 and 8 servings of a dairy product, and because such products are commonly shunned by weight-conscious teenaged girls, many in this age group have inadequate intakes and may require supplementation. Of the calcium salts, calcium carbonate is preferable because 40% of its calcium is available for absorption. Tums-Ex is a convenient and inexpensive source of supplementary calcium. The need for supplementary calcium is more acute in the adolescent female who is amenorrheic, either as a result of anorexia nervosa or athletic involvement, because of the increased risk of osteoporosis.

Zinc Deficiency

In teenaged females who have become true vegetarians or who have placed themselves on starvation diets, the risk of zinc deficiency exists. Zinc is generally found in protein, and its deficiency may result in a variety of sequelae, including hair loss, dry skin, loss of discriminatory taste perception, and pubertal delay. Vegan diets, those that exclude all animal foods, are low in vitamins B6, B12, riboflavin, calcium, and iron, as well as zinc. A diet for vegetarians and vegans is found in Table 8. Secondary zinc deficiency occurs in abusers of alcohol, in whom excretion of zinc is increased.

Vitamin Deficiencies

Adolescents' intake of vitamins A, B6, C, and folacin are generally below recommended levels. In addition, intake of vitamins B6, B12, and riboflavin, may be inadequate in vegan adolescents. These same vitamins are low in association with use of oral contraceptives, which may lower levels of vitamin C, folacin, and pyridoxine while raising levels of vitamin A. Smoking is also associated with lowered levels of vitamin C. A diet consisting of 100 mg daily is now recommended for smokers. Alcohol abusers experience impaired absorption of folacin by mucosal cells of the small intestine, and long-term abuse reduces hepatic stores of vitamin A.

Nutrition of Pregnant Adolescents

In recognition of the increased needs for iron during pregnancy, recommendations have recently been increased to 30 mg daily by a committee of the National Academy of Science. Calcium and protein needs are also elevated during pregnancy.

Dietary Excesses

In addition to deficiency diseases, adolescents are at risk for diseases of dietary excess, such as "reactive" obesity (see p.141), which typically begins during adolescence. For another example, ingestion of excessive amounts of

TABLE 8. Food Guide for the Pregnant Adolescent and the Adolescent Consuming a Mixed Protein, Lacto-Ovo-Vegetarian, or Vegan Diet

	Number of Servings for Type of Diet			
	Mixed		*Lacto-ovo-vegetarian*	*Vegan*
Food Group	Nonpregnant Adolescent	Pregnant Adolescent	Nonpregnant Adolescent	Nonpregnant Adolescent
Milk and Milk Products	4	6	4	0
Protein Foods				
Animal sources	2	2	0	0
Legumes	1	1	2	3
Nuts	1	1	1	2
Fruits and Vegetables				
Vitamin C-rich	1	1	2	2
Dark green	1	1	1	3
Other	2	2	3	1
Whole Grain Cereal Products	4	4	6	6
Fats and Oils	2	2	2	2

Adapted from King JC, Cohenour SH, Corruccini CG, Schneeman P: Evaluation and modification of the basic four food guide. J Nutr Ed, 10:27, 1978.

certain vitamins, such as vitamin A, often prescribed for the treatment of acne, may result in complications such as hair loss, pseudotumor cerebri, hepatosplenomegaly, fissuring at the corners of the mouth, desquamation of palms and soles, and anorexia.

A dietary history should be taken from every adolescent patient in order to discover and possibly prevent nutritional problems, as well as their psychosocial ramifications (see pp. 129–141).

Growth and Development

ISSUES

1. Has puberty begun at the appropriate time?
2. If not, should an evaluation be undertaken?
3. Has the patient been adequately prepared for his or her pubertal development?
4. Does the patient have any concerns about it?
5. What changes have occurred as a result of onset of puberty: in diet, in familial interaction, in peer relationships and in other aspects of life?

The physical growth of the second decade of life is the most dramatic of any throughout the life cycle, involving major changes that are both quantitative and qualitative. During adolescence, most individuals double their prepubertal growth in one quarter of the time. The skeletal growth spurt, increases in muscular tissue in males and in fat in females, and the development of reproductive organs and secondary sex characteristics are unique to adolescence. These events form the script for the physician's assessment of physical growth of the teenager.

FAMILY HISTORY

Because patterns of growth are similar among members of the same family, particularly between mothers and their children of either sex, the family history provides the single best reference standard for assessing an individual adolescent's growth. The history of physical growth and development may fruitfully begin with recording the family history of these events. Obtaining the history of parents' pubertal growth and development in the teenager's presence often has the added advantage of providing him or her with reassuring information (for example, the short 15-year-old's learning that his 6′5″ father didn't have a growth spurt until 16 years of age). The finding of delay in development or difference in growth in the adolescent when compared with that of the parents should signal the possibility of pathology and the need for an evaluation, even if the teenager falls within the population norms for the event under consideration.

Early identification of the teenager with primary amenorrhea is desirable in terms of her self-image and sense of sexual adequacy, and in order to decrease potentially adverse medical sequelae (see pp. 103–114). For example, the mean age for menarche is currently 12.4 years in the U.S., with a range of 10–16 years. That notwithstanding, a 14-year-old girl who is premenarcheal may require evaluation for primary amenorrhea if her mother's age of menarche was 11 years, because of the close correlation between mother's and daughter's menarcheal age. The correlation between siblings is even higher, so that the age of menarche of the patient's sisters provides even a better reference standard than that of her mother. Stated somewhat differently, the average difference in age at menarche between sisters is 13 months, for fraternal twins 10 months, and for identical twins reared together less than 3 months. Any female teenager who has not menstruated within 2 years of the age of menarche of her sister or mother, or who is over 16 years should undergo evaluation. Regardless of age, the patient who has completed stage 4 of development of secondary sex characteristics or in whom more than 2 years have elapsed since breast budding, and menarche has not started, should be evaluated. The content of the evaluation is found on page 112.

PREPUBERTAL GROWTH

After the family history of growth is determined, historical data about earlier childhood growth of the patient is obtained, if not already part of the medical record. By the age of 10 years (that is, prior to the pubertal growth spurt), females have reached approximately 85% of their ultimate height, and males more than 75% of theirs. By age 10, slightly more than half of adult weight has been achieved. Even more importantly, patterns of growth have been established prior to puberty, such that those destined to be early maturers already have advanced growth curves. Girls with early menarche (before 13 years) are taller and weigh more at ages 6 through 8 years than those whose menarche occurs after 13 years of age. The same relationships have long been observed for boys, such that those who were tall as children generally enter puberty earlier than those who were shorter. During the childhood years there is actually a slight deceleration in the height velocity curve, because the rate of growth from each year to the next is slightly less (averaging 5–6 cm/yr). This rate is the same for males and females.

HEIGHT AND SKELETAL GROWTH

At the peak of the height spurt, males grow an average rate of 10 cm per year (10.3 ± 1.5 cm/yr) and females about 8 cm per year (9.0 ± 1.0 cm/yr.). The mean age for this growth spurt is 14 years (range, 12–17 years) for males and 12 years (10.5–13 years) for females at a sex maturity rating (SMR) of 3 or 4 in both sexes. The earlier the growth spurt, the greater its velocity; the later, the taller the individual ultimately.

The pattern of acceleration of linear growth throughout the body is also fairly predictable.[63] The first body part to elongate (and also the first to cease growing) is the foot (Fig. 1). Because of the high price of shoes, parents can provide accurate historical information about this growth parameter ("Ah yes, last year he outgrew his sneakers three times before even wearing them out!"). Approximately 6 months after onset of accelerated foot growth, there is elongation of the calf, followed by the thigh. Similarly, in the upper limb, distal bones elongate before those more proximal. The resultant transient disproportion in hand and foot size contributes to the clumsiness that often characterizes teenagers. Approximately 4 months after the peak of leg-length growth, the hips and chest broaden, the latter more so in males than females. The trunk lengthens and chest deepens last in the usual progression.

SEX DIFFERENCES IN PUBERTAL GROWTH PATTERNS

In contrast with the situation in childhood, characterized by similar growth rates and patterns in males and females, important sex differences in growth emerge during puberty, some of which have already been noted: the earlier and smaller growth spurt in females; longer legs in males as a result of a protracted period of prepubertal growth; and increased bi-acromial width in males. Adult contour differences arise because of the greater spurt in shoulder width and chest breadth among males and increased hip width of females during puberty, owing to the effects of androgens and estrogens, respectively. Female fat accumulation during puberty also contributes to increased hip width. The legs and arms of males are longer than those of females relative to total body length because of later onset of the growth spurt in females. The carrying angle of the male's arm is less than that of the female, a phenomenon explained by differential pubertal growth of cartilage at the lateral humeral epicondyle between the sexes. Approximately 4 months after leg-length acceleration peaks, the cranial bones undergo a growth spurt. As a result, the jaw becomes more prominent, especially in males. The hyoid bone lowers as a result of elongation of the pharynx.

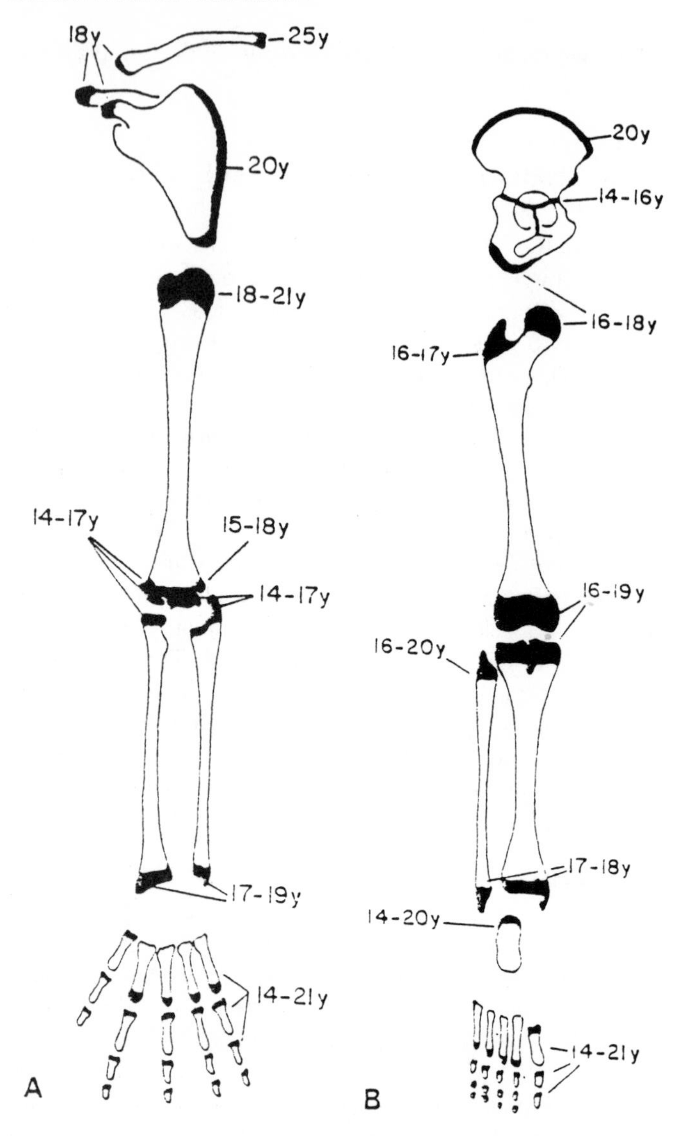

FIGURE 1. Ages of physical closure of epiphyses. A = arm; B = leg. (From Ogden JA: Skeletal Injury in the Child. Philadelphia, Lea and Febiger, 1982, pp 56–57, with permission.)

DENTAL DEVELOPMENT

The canines and first molars of the primary dentition are shed prior to puberty. At this time, the permanent cuspids and first and second premolars erupt. A close (r = 0.62) correlation has been found between the age of menarche and age of alveolar eruption of the second molars. The "wisdom teeth" (third molars) erupt during later adolescence. The observation that dental development patterns of late childhood predict the timing of the adolescent height spurt, pubic hair growth, and menarche further suggests that dental age assessment may provide an additional means for anticipating adolescent growth patterns.

WEIGHT GROWTH

There are prominent sex differences in the pubertal growth of soft tissues. Both sexes experience a marked weight gain during puberty, nearly doubling prepubertal weight within the few years of onset of the weight spurt. The peak of this spurt tends to occur about 6 months after that of the height spurt. The pubertal increase in weight in males is largely accounted for by the increase in muscle mass. There is a fourfold greater increase in number of muscle cells in males than in females during puberty. The peak in muscle strength is noted approximately 14 months after the peak of the height velocity curve, and corresponds to SMR 4. During puberty in females, fat increases from approximately 8% to 20% of total body composition.

VARIATIONS IN GROWTH

Normal pubertal changes in height and weight, particularly if they occur at a rate different from that of the peer group, often give rise to concerns that should be detected and addressed during the well adolescent visit. In the National Health Examination Survey (Cycle 3), a national probability sample, 49% of 12- and 13-year-old males wanted to be taller. In addition to dissatisfaction with height, 73% of the 12- to 17-year-old male sample wished they were more muscular. Of 12- to 17-year-old females in this survey, 37–60% were dissatisfied with their weights and desired to be thinner.[19] The desire for thinness bore little relationship to actual fatness, in contrast to the adolescent males. When desire to be thinner was examined in relationship to stage of pubertal development by Gross et al., it was found that advancing pubertal development was correlated with increasing dissatisfaction with weight among females. This dissatisfaction also correlated with socioeconomic status, with greater dissatisfaction being found in those from higher socioeconomic status group. This observation suggests that the normal events of pubertal development are viewed by the majority of females as negative.

In a recent study of adolescents in an upper-middle class community,[12] 65% of young females (12-year-olds) expressed dissatisfaction with weight, an increase of 30% over a similar study 15 years earlier. The additional finding that 45% of 12-year-old girls wanted to be more muscular also suggests a change in their perception of the idealized female body. In a more recent study, Killen et al.[23] found that 33% of tenth-grade females judged themselves to be overweight. As a result, dieting among young adolescent girls has become common—about 33% of all adolescent females report dieting, 10% total fasting, 10% purging, and 18% use of diet pills.

GROWTH OF REPRODUCTIVE ORGANS AND SECONDARY SEX CHARACTERISTICS

The most impressive of all physical changes of puberty involve the development of reproductive capability and secondary sex characteristics. Although the source of the signal for stimulation of appropriate releasing and inhibiting of hormones of the hypothalamus, which triggers pubertal development, is yet to be elucidated, much is now known about the functional interrelationships between organs in the hypothalamic-pituitary-gonadal axis that are responsible for these events. As the time for puberty nears, the hypothalamus is believed to decrease its sensitivity to circulating levels of gonadal hormones. Luteinizing hormone–releasing hormone (LHRH) is then produced by the arcuate nucleus of the hypothalamus in a pulsatile fashion that stimulates pituitary gonadotropin production, particularly during sleep. These hormones then stimulate their target organs, either testes or ovaries, to produce testosterone or estrogen, respectively. Testosterone and estrogen are responsible for the growth of reproductive organs and the development of secondary sex characteristics.

TABLE 9. Dimensions of Testicular Volume Standards of Prader Orchiometer*

Standard Volume	Smallest Dimension (cm)	Largest Dimension (cm)
1	1.0	1.6
2	1.3	2.0
3	1.5	2.4
4	1.7	2.6
5	1.8	2.7
6	1.9	2.8
8	2.1	3.1
10	2.2	3.5
12	2.4	3.8
15	2.6	4.1
20	3.9	4.3
25	4.1	4.8

From Friedman IM, Goldberg E: Reference materials for the practice of adolescent medicine. Pediatr Clin North Am 27:193–209, 1980, with permission.

*Measured by authors with Harpenden skinfold calipers.

TABLE 10. Development of Male Genitalia During Puberty

Stage 1:	Childhood size and configuration of genitalia.
Stage 2:	Enlargement of testes and scrotum, the latter reddening and thinning.
Stage 3:	Lengthening of penis, associated with further enlargement of testes and scrotum.
Stage 4:	Widening as well as further lengthening of penis. Further enlargement of testes and scrotum, and deepening pigmentation of scrotal skin.
Stage 5:	Adult configuration and size of genitalia.

During puberty, testes grow from their childlike volume of approximately 2 cc to adult size of approximately 25 cc (Table 9). The initial increase in size is primarily the result of an increase in size of the seminiferous tubules. Within the 2 years following the onset of growth of the seminiferous tubules, Sertoli cells and spermatogonia become differentiated and multiply, further contributing to testicular size. Development of testosterone-secreting Leydig cells lags behind that of tubule cells, explaining why testicular enlargement is noted before the growth of the penis. The epididymis, seminal vesicles, and prostate enlarge as well. Development of the male genitalia progresses in an orderly sequence, as described first by Greulich[17] and later by Tanner[63] (Table 10 and Fig. 2).

On the average, it takes approximately 2 years to pass from the second to fourth stage (SMR 2–4) and another 2 years to reach stage 5 (SMR 5).

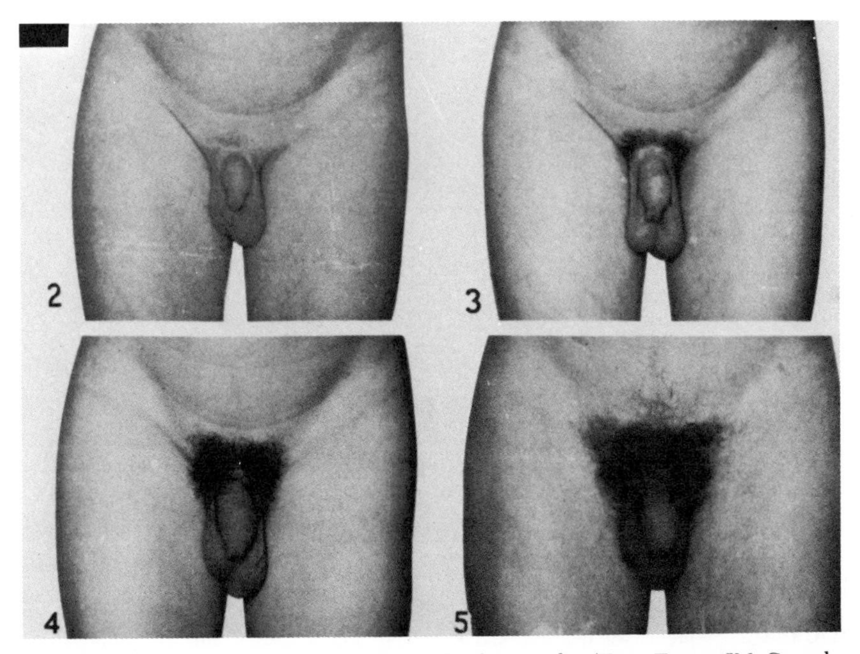

FIGURE 2. Pubertal development in size of male genitalia. (From Tanner JM: Growth at Adolescence, 2nd ed. Oxford, Blackwell Scientific Publications, Ltd., 1962, with permission.)

TABLE 11. Development of Pubic Hair in Males During Puberty

PH Stage 1:	Prepubertal—no pubic hair.
PH Stage 2:	Sparse downy hair at base of phallus.
PH Stage 3:	Darkening, coarsening, curling of hair, which extends upward and laterally.
PH Stage 4:	Hair of adult consistency limited to the mons.
PH Stage 5:	Hair spreads to medial aspect of thighs.

Normal variations in penile size often prove to be of concern to the young male adolescent. Reassurance offered should be based on knowledge of stages of growth of the genitalia (i.e., if he is not yet at stage 5 there will be additional growth), as well as on the fact that differences in size of the penis in the flaccid state are minimized when the penis is erect. The use of photographs of normal progression of development is helpful, remembering to explain differences between uncircumcised and circumcised penises. Synchronous with development of the male genitalia during puberty is progression of growth of pubic hair, which begins slightly later, typically between stages (SMR) 3 and 4. This progression involves texture, consistency, and distribution of hair from downy to silky to coarse and from the base of the phallus laterally (Table 11).

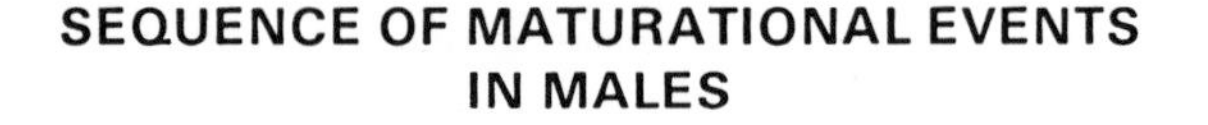

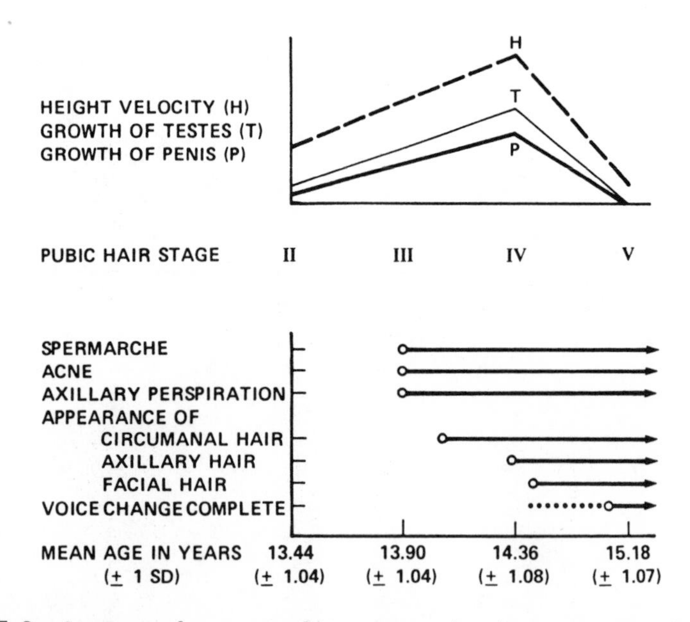

FIGURE 3. Sequence of maturational events in males. (From Litt IF: Adolescent development. In Behrman RE, Vaughan VC III (eds): Nelson Textbook of Pediatrics, 13th ed. Philadelphia, W.B. Saunders, 1987, with permission.)

Completion of this developmental sequence takes an average of 4 years. Development of pubic hair and genitalia typically proceeds within 1–2 stages of each other (Fig. 3).

Approximately 1 year after onset of testicular growth, and closely related in time to appearance of pubic hair (SMR 2), most males experience ejaculation, a dramatic event that clearly differentiates pubertal orgasm from that which preceded it in childhood, as well as from female orgasm. Contrary to the popular notion that nocturnal emission marks the onset of ejaculatory experience, two-thirds of the Kinsey sample[24] reported ejaculation through masturbation to have been the first event, with nocturnal emission occurring approximately 1 year later. The ejaculate is composed largely of secretions from the prostate, which grows during puberty, and, to a lesser extent, from the seminal vesicles and sperm.

Spermarche occurs before the peak of the height velocity curve at any stage from SMR 1–5. The medium age for appearance of sperm in the first morning urine sample is 13.5–14.5 years in different studies. Although complete reproductive maturity is not reached until SMR 5, those data suggest that impregnation is possible at an earlier stage.

Other Secondary Sex Characteristics

Facial and body hair appear during puberty under the stimulation of androgen secretion. The timing and progression of these events are so variable that no consistent schema, such as that used for pubic hair or genitalia development, is feasible. Axillary hair typically appears approximately when pubic hair is at stage 4, is usually preceded by circumanal hair, and is associated with appearance of facial hair. Facial hair begins at the corners of the upper lip and spreads medially. Growth of hair on the chin, the beard, is the last event of facial hair growth and usually follows completion of pubic hair, stage 5. Chest hair is also a late event, appearing last in the sequence of body hair growth. The typical sequence of hair development is outlined below:

Pubic hair (Stage 4)
Axillary hair
Facial hair
- Upper lip
  Spreads medially from corner
- Upper cheek
- Under lower lip
- Chin

Chest hair

The effect of testosterone on stimulation of growth of cartilage cells of the thyroid and cricoid cartilage and of laryngeal muscles is responsible for the gradual, yet often unpredictable, deepening of voice that occurs during male puberty.

At the time of appearance of axillary hair, the apocrine sweat glands become functional, causing body odor, another frequent concern of the self-conscious adolescent.

Gynecomastia

Gynecomastia, enlargement of the male breast, includes projection of the areola and the appearance of a firm mass below. It is a common pubertal event, occurring in approximately 40% of males. It typically occurs about the time that the genitalia have reached SMR stage 4 of development and persists for an average of 1½ years. Gynecomastia is most likely caused by estrogen stimulation, but there is no evidence of hormonal differences between those with and without this condition. Gynecomastia is more commonly bilateral than unilateral and occurs in thin as well as obese boys. Because adolescents with gynecomastia are often concerned about the presence of breasts, it is wise to offer reassurance, regardless of whether the patient has raised questions about it. One approach is to inquire about it before actual examination, prefacing the question with a statement such as: "Since nearly half of all *normal* teenage boys experience some growth of their breasts for a year or two during their normal pubertal development, I thought you might have some questions about this." If not addressed, concern about having breasts may manifest itself in refusal to attend gym class, because of its implications for public undressing, or occasionally truancy from school. The physician should consider embarrassment about gynecomastia as a possible explanation when a teenage male with minimal findings on physical examination requests an excuse from gym class following a minor injury. A discussion of the matter will prove reassuring to the boy with gynecomastia who may be harboring doubts about his masculinity or may be helpful in preventing the patient without gynecomastia from teasing his less fortunate classmate. It is rare that gynecomastia persists into adulthood or is of sufficient magnitude to justify reduction mammoplasty. Rare pathologic causes of gynecomastia are listed in Table 12.

Acne

As a dermatologic problem, acne is discussed fully later in the book (see pp. 87–88), but it is mentioned here in the context of secondary sex characteristics because of its origins. Increase in testosterone at the time of puberty in both sexes, and more specifically its metabolite dihydrotestosterone, is responsible for enlargement of sebaceous follicles and stimulation of secretion of sebum. Sebum is converted to free fatty acids by *Corynebacterium acnes* (Fig. 4), and causes irritation and follicle blockage, the forerunners of the lesions of acne. Acne can be classified according to

TABLE 12. Disorders Associated with Gynecomastia

Klinefelter syndrome
Traumatic paraplegia
Male pseudohermaphroditism
Testicular feminization syndrome
Reifenstein syndrome
17-Ketosteroid reductase deficiency
Endocrine tumors (seminoma, Leydig cell tumor, teratoma, feminizing adrenal tumor, hepatoma, leukemia, hemophilia, bronchogenic carcinoma, leprosy, etc.)
Hypothyroidism
Hyperthyroidism
Cirrhosis
Herpes zoster
Friedreich ataxia

gradations of severity (Table 13). There are no temporal relationships between stages, and most adolescents never reach the most advanced stage.

Development of secondary sex characteristics in females reflects increasing levels of estrogen and androgens throughout puberty (breast, reproductive tract and hair, apocrine and sweat glands). The effects of androgens on the development and progression of pubic and axillary hair are identical to those of males (Table 14 and Fig. 5). The extent to which facial or body hair will appear during puberty is largely genetically determined, unless a pathogenic masculinizing condition exists. Estrogens are responsible for breast development, which follows an orderly sequence (Table 15 and Fig. 6).

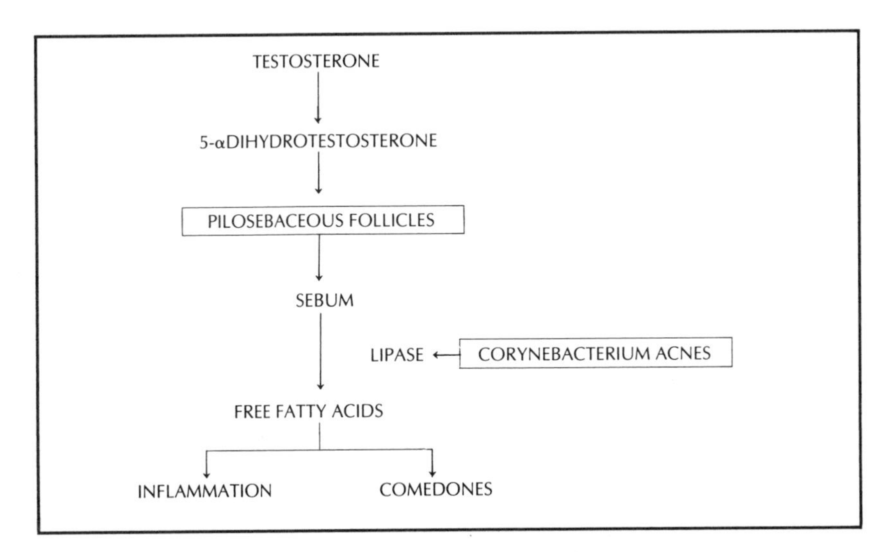

FIGURE 4. Pathogenesis of acne.

TABLE 13. Classification of Acne

Grade 1:	Comedones
Grade 2:	Comedones and superficial pustular and inflammatory lesions confined to the face
Grade 3:	Comedones, small pustules, deeper inflamed lesions of the face, neck, tops of shoulders, and presternal region
Grade 4:	Extensive cystic acne

From Pillsbury DM, Shelley WB, Kligman AM: A Manual of Cutaneous Medicine. Philadelphia, W.B. Saunders Co., 1961, with permission.

Stage 2 breast development (SMR 2 B) is usually the first sign of puberty in females and there is a close relationship between pubic hair and breast stages thereafter (Fig. 7). Seventy-five percent of females pass through all stages; in the remainder, stage 4 may be skipped.

Both internal and external genitalia also develop under the influence of estrogen, but the gradual nature of changes and individual variability have heretofore precluded their usefulness in a staging system.

At about the time of breast budding (stage 2), the vaginal mucosa begins to lose its red, glistening appearance and becomes dull and pink as a result of estrogen-induced thickening of vaginal epithelium and increased deposition of glycogen within these epithelial cells. These changes have implications for the vaginal microflora, rendering the vaginal mucosa more resistant to bacterial penetration, favoring appearance of Döderlein (lactic acid–forming) bacteria, and increasing susceptibility to growth of yeast. A change to an acid pH (4–5) naturally follows. The labia minora become increasingly pigmented and eroticised, as does the clitoris, which enlarges slightly.

The ovaries, the source of estrogen, enlarge about a year before the stage of breast budding (stage 2) under pulsatile stimulation by pituitary gonadotropins. In contrast to male gonads, however, there is no increase in number of gametes during puberty. The uterus increases in size during puberty, with the fundus enlarging more than the cervix. The endometrium thickens and differentiates, and the myometrium increases in size and in cellular content of actinomysin, creatinine kinase (CK), and adenosine triphosphate (ATP). The former occurs as a prerequisite to menses and the latter permits the contractility necessary for childbirth and is associated with menstrual cramps.

TABLE 14. Stages of Development of Pubic Hair During Female Puberty

PH Stage 1:	Prepubertal—no pubic hair
PH Stage 2:	Sparse downy hair at medial aspect of labia majora
PH Stage 3:	Darkening, coarsening, curling of hair, which extends upward and laterally
PH Stage 4:	Hair of adult consistency limited to the mons
PH Stage 5:	Hair spreads to medial aspect of thighs

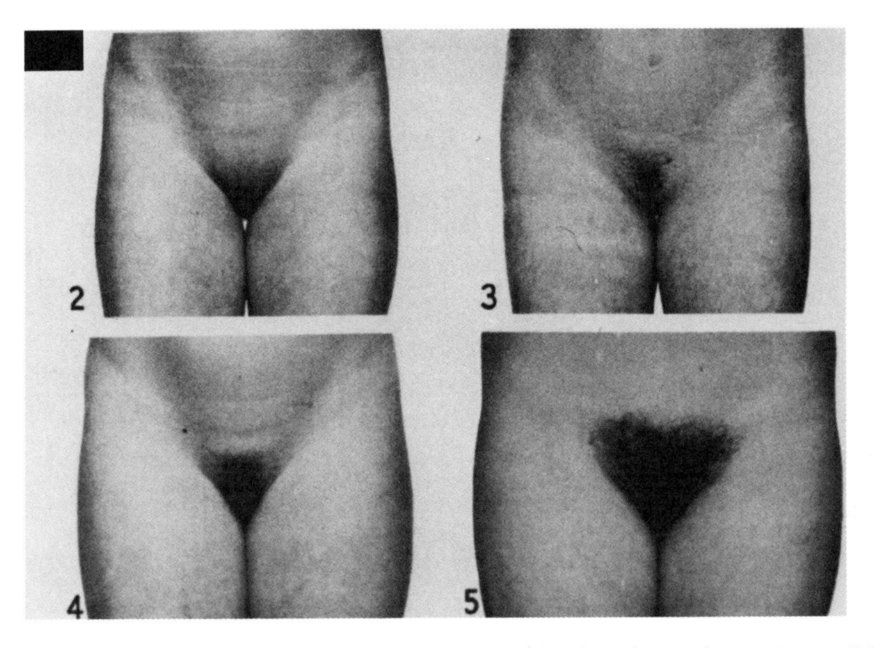

FIGURE 5. Development of pubic hair during female puberty. (From Tanner JM: Growth at Adolescence, 2nd ed. Oxford, Blackwell Scientific Publications, Ltd., 1962, with permission.)

Menarche

Menarche is the most dramatic event of female puberty and occurs at a predictable time in relationship to other pubertal changes (Fig. 7). Ten percent of females have menarche at stage 2 breast development, 20% at stage 3, 60% at stage 4, and 10% at stage 5. Menarche tends to occur just after the peak of the height velocity curve (r = 0.93) and coincides with the peak of the weight velocity curve. The physician should ascertain whether

TABLE 15. Stages of Development of the Breast During Female Puberty

(B) Stage 1:	Prepubertal—no breast tissue
(B) Stage 2:	Appearance of a breast bud
(B) Stage 3:	Enlargement of breast and areola
(B) Stage 4:	Areola and nipple form a mound atop underlying breast tissue
(B) Stage 5:	Adult configuration, with areola and breast having smooth contour

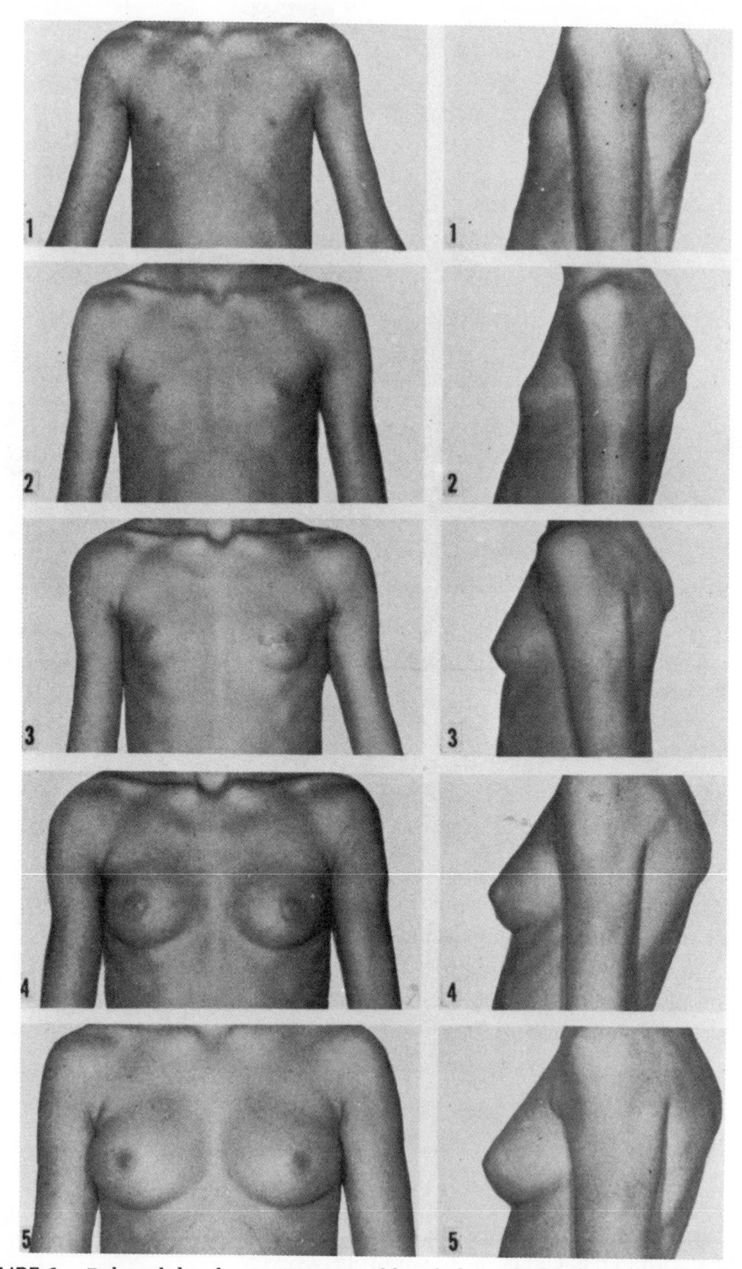

FIGURE 6. Pubertal development in size of female breasts. (From Tanner JM: Growth at Adolescence, 2nd ed. Oxford, Blackwell Scientific Publications, Ltd., 1962, with permission.)

SEQUENCE OF MATURATIONAL EVENTS IN FEMALES

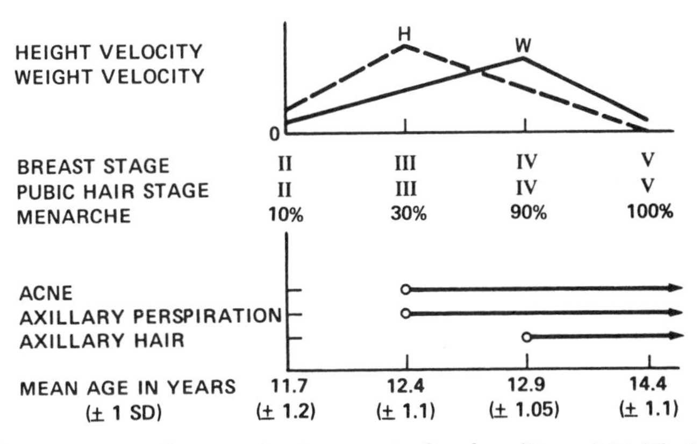

FIGURE 7. Sequence of maturational events in females. (From Litt IF: Adolescent development. In Behrman RE, Vaughan VC III (eds): Nelson Textbook of Pediatrics, 13th ed. Philadelphia, W.B. Saunders, 1987, with permission.)

menarche has yet occurred and, if not, determine whether evaluation is necessary, remembering that the best reference standard for an individual is her mother's and sister's age of menarche. If evaluation is indicated, reassurance about the patient's normality should be stressed and information about pubertal development provided.

Bone Age

X-ray determination of the course of development of individual bones and the number of centers of ossification by comparison to a set of standards (Fig. 8) allows for assessment of skeletel (bone) age. The hand and wrist (left) are typically chosen for study. Separate standards are available for males and females because of the greater maturity of females at all ages. According to Tanner, "males are on average between 75% and 80% of the skeletal age of females of the same chronological age." Sex differences, race, socioeconomic status, and physique also appear to influence skeletal age. Because standards commonly used are based on chronologic age, the standard deviation of hand skeletal age calculations increase to 12 months at puberty. Bone age appears to be fairly consistent, so that those who become early pubertal maturers have had advanced bone ages during childhood. Of all measures of pubertal growth, bone age is related most closely to age of appearance of secondary sex characteristics (for example, the correlation between menarche and the Todd skeletal age at age 13 is -0.85).

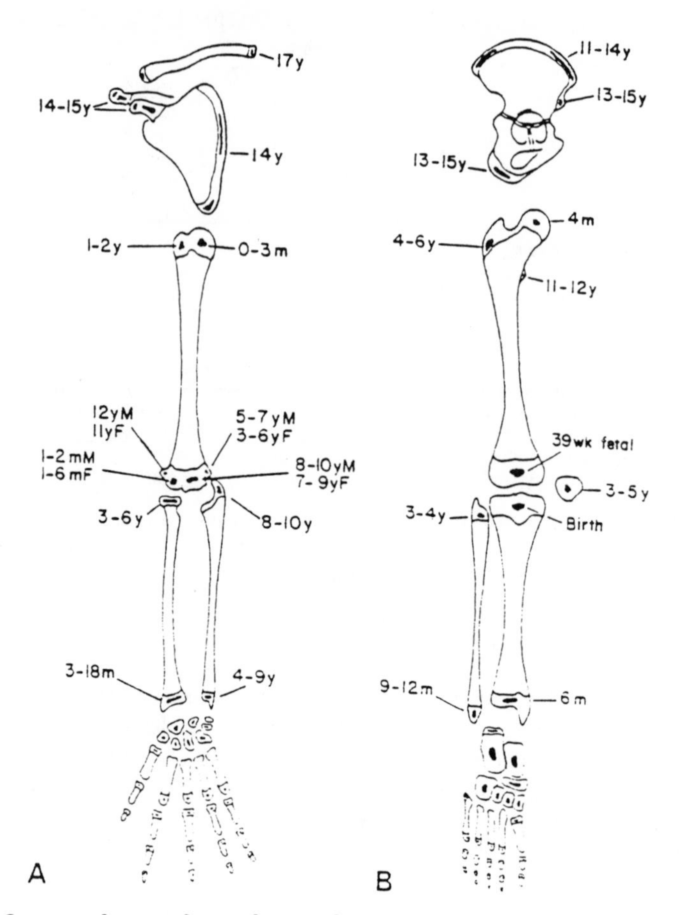

FIGURE 8. Age of onset of secondary ossification centers. A = arm; B = leg. (From Ogden JA: Skeletal Injury in the Child. Philadelphia, Lea and Febiger, 1982, pp 56–57, with permission.)

Dental Age

Standards exist for the timing of eruption of each tooth.[18] Comparison with such standards yields a dental age. Because almost all teeth have calcified or erupted before puberty, dental age is of less value during adolescence than during earlier years.

Review of Systems

PSYCHIATRIC EVALUATION

Mental Status Examination

The gross state of psychological functioning of an adolescent patient may be appraised by performance of the mental status examination. A formal assessment of this kind is, however, often embarrassing and demeaning to the teenager, and it is preferable to evaluate the domains delineated below in the context of the interview and by observation whenever possible. It is also important to consider possible cultural and experiential aspects of the patient's behavior before concluding that there is a mental status abnormality (for example, hallucinations may be experienced in the context of certain religious settings, and failure to make eye contact may be culturally determined). The first component of the evaluation is assessment of the organization of the adolescent's dress, manner of relating, general level of activity, and presence of unusual body movement, such as tics.

Orientation. Is the sensorium clear?; is the patient confused or unaware of where he or she is? (place); time of day?, month?, year?, or who he or she is? Gross abnormalities of this kind are most often caused by intoxication from drugs or alcohol, or by head trauma, or occur postictally in the adolescent patient.

Speech/Language. The intent of this portion of the examination is to assess the adolescent's ability to communicate (how understandable and articulate he or she is). Speech is generally divided into expressive (talking) and receptive (understanding) components. A defect in either is referred to as aphasia. **Broca aphasia** describes inability to speak or speaking in a telegraphic fashion. Patients with such a defect usually can understand and follow verbal commands. In **receptive aphasia,** the patient is able to speak but the words are meaningless (neologisms). In both types of aphasia, the patient is able to repeat individual words verbatim. Aphasia in the adolescent usually signals the presence of a lesion in the dominant temporal lobe.

Memory. Short-term (recent) memory is the most vulnerable to disruption from use of alcohol or drugs, or from head trauma or organic brain disease. This is tested by having the patient repeat, five minutes after hearing them, four or five unrelated words that describe objects. A less threatening approach is to ask the patient to tell you what he or she had to eat at the most recent meal.

In the course of taking a typical medical history, the patient is required to relate events in the past. This is usually sufficient for the purposes of evaluating remote (long-term) memory.

Intellect. This component of the evaluation is heavily dependent upon the patient's level of cognitive development. Most adolescents do not achieve the capacity for abstract thinking until late adolescence. Moreover, any anxious or shy patient may have difficulty with this component of the examination. The ability to think abstractly is typically tested by having the patient interpret proverbs (for example, "The early bird catches the worm"; "People in glass houses shouldn't throw stones") and to describe similarities and differences between words. Another method of informal assessment of intellect involves testing of arithmetic ability by asking the patient to count. This is best achieved with the adolescent by presenting a practical problem that requires multiplication or division for solution: "I will give you enough pills for a month. At three a day, how many should that be?"

Thought. This component of the mental status examination evaluates ability to differentiate reality from fantasy, reasoning ability, and logic. The existence of hallucinations, delusions, looseness of associations, and presence of obsessive or bizarre thoughts are investigated. In the context of routine history taking, the adolescent female who is sexually active may be asked why she thinks she has not yet gotten pregnant. Or the youngster who has had an illness may be asked why he or she thinks he or she got sick. Although responses may or may not be physiologically or epidemiologically correct, they will provide insight into the patient's thought processing. Abnormalities in this domain may suggest schizophrenia, chronic drug use, mental retardation, or developmental delay. They require further assessment by a mental health professional.

Emotionality. The fact that normal adolescents may experience strong emotions and undergo fairly extreme mood changes should be kept in mind, lest criteria established for adults be applied inappropriately and the teenager be misdiagnosed as having a mood disorder.

Depression. The high suicide rate during adolescence mandates that the health professional pay close attention to the finding of depressed affect in the adolescent patient (see pp. 164–168 for a more complete discussion).

Appropriateness of the Expressed Emotion in the Context of the Teenager's History. When the patient describes excruciating pain with a matter-of-fact expression on his or her face, "la belle indifférence," it is suggestive of the possibility of a conversion reaction.

Feelings of Depersonalization. Although such feelings occur in schizophrenia and drug intoxications, they may be normal if they occur occasionally in the otherwise normal adolescent.

Perceptual and Motor Capacities. This component assesses the patient's coordination, motor skills, attention span, and capacity for understanding and reproducing symbols in drawing and writing. This is most important in the assessment of the younger child, but a previously unevaluated adolescent with an attention deficit disorder or an adolescent under the influence of drugs may be found to have abnormalities in this area as well.

Evaluation for a Possible Learning Disability

Although it is rare for youngsters with a learning disability to reach adolescence before the problem is identified, teenagers from medically underserved areas may have escaped earlier detection. By the time adolescence is reached, there may be compensatory or avoidant behaviors or those acquired to disguise the learning disability, as well as adverse sequelae such as delinquency, school avoidance or school failure, all of which may make diagnosis and treatment difficult. Screening may be begun by having the teenager write out his or her daily school schedule. This permits rapid assessment of writing skills, such as sequencing, letter reversals, memory, and spelling. Providing the patient with numbers that have relevance to him or her, such as height and weight along with metric conversion factors, will permit observation of simply arithmetic skills. A more comprehensive assessment is accomplished through use of standardized instruments, such as those developed by Levine (Adolescent Age Group Form for Functional and Developmental Assessment).[21] Signs of neuromaturational delay include those of gross motor function, fine motor function, visual-spatial orientation, temporal-sequential organization, language, memory, and behavioral and stylistic observations. As helpful as this assessment is in the younger child, it and other standardized tests for learning disabilities are much less useful during adolescence because of the "ceiling out" effect during the preadolescent years.

NEUROLOGIC EVALUATION

Deterioration in school performance, irritability, or emotional lability will suggest cerebral dysfunction, the result of increased intracranial pressure (secondary to a tumor or pseudotumor cerebri), depression, or drug abuse.

Vertigo, the sensation of the room tilting or spinning, may result from diseases of the inner ear or the effect of drugs.

Syncope may result from a cardiac arrhythmia, postural hypotension (as is common in anorexia nervosa), or the effect of drugs, either prescribed (such as tricyclic antidepressants) or illicit.

Headache. The diagnosis is based on the knowledge of the quality, location, and chronology of the pain and the presence or absence of associated symptoms. (See pp. 115–118 for a differential diagnosis of headaches in the adolescent.)

Seizures. Temporal lobe and photosensitive epilepsy may begin during adolescence. The onset of other seizure disorders during adolescence is, however, rare and suggests the possibility of prior traumatic injury to the brain, a tumor, or drug overdose or withdrawal (see pp. 160–163). In females with preexisting grand mal epilepsy, the frequency of seizures may be increased in the premenstrual phase of the cycle.

Adolescents with epilepsy, regardless of their age at onset, often encounter psychological difficulty resulting from being different from the peer group, not feeling in control of one's own body, needing to take medication, and not being able to drive a car. As a result, some teenagers with epilepsy may become depressed or noncompliant with medication, or develop "pseudo-seizures."

HEAD, EYES, EARS NOSE, AND THROAT (HEENT)

Head

Hair. **Hair style** is often a statement made by the young person about who he or she is or would like to be. It is often the symbol of rebellion against parental authority or of identification with a particular peer culture, and thus may provide useful information about the adolescent's stage of psychosocial development.

Hair loss (alopecia) may result from hypothyroidism, fungal infections, traction associated with certain hairstyles (cornrows), mannerisms (twirling hair), emotional distress (trichotillomania), or nutritional deficiency (zinc deficiency from anorexia nervosa). It may be localized or generalized (alopecia totalis). Hair loss is a distressing problem with many possible causes. A careful history will assist in determining its etiology, which will facilitate treatment.

It is first necessary to ascertain whether the hair is coming out at the root or breaking along the shaft. The latter suggests that trichotillomania or hair style may be responsible. In both conditions, the hair breaks as a result of twisting, pulling, or traction. Braiding or cornrows, currently popular with teenagers, may predispose to this problem. Hair loss from the root has a broader differential diagnosis in the adolescent, including nutritional, endocrine, infectious, autoimmune, dermatologic, and toxic etiologies. Among the nutritional causes to be considered in the adolescent are rapid weight loss and hypervitaminosis A, both of which cause conversion of an excessive number of hairs from the growing (anagen) to resting (telogen) phase. Hairs in the resting phase fall out approximately 100 days later, in contrast to those in the growing phase, which last approximately 1000 days. Acquired hypothyroidism may cause loss of anagen hairs, as does chemotherapeutic agents and radiation. When hair loss is associated with itching, fungal infection should be suspected. Alopecia areata, thought to be an autoimmune phenomenon, is typically asymptomatic and causes sharply demarcated, smooth, hairless round or oval patches. Naturally, congenital causes of hair loss do not have to be considered in this age group, as they must in the younger child. On the other hand, late adolescence is the time when one first sees male pattern baldness (androgenic alopecia), which is the most common cause of hair loss in males in this age group. These patients experience a gradual thinning of hair over the occiput and lateral frontal hairline after completion of pubertal development, have a positive family history, and have no other symptoms.

Infestations. Lice (pediculosis) may be caused by close bodily contact or sharing of hair brushes or combs, a common adolescent activity.

Suboccipital Lymphadenopathy. Infectious mononucleosis (EBV) is the most common cause in the adolescent. Cytomegalovirus should also be considered in the differential diagnosis, as should Hodgkin disease. Scrofula is one of the most common manifestations of tuberculosis in the adolescent. In the intravenous drug-using or sexually promiscuous adolescent, the finding of lymphadenopathy at any location should raise concern about the possibility of AIDS.

Sinuses

Pain over the sinuses, typically the frontal and maxillary, associated with asymmetry in transillumination, should suggest sinusitis. Because the frontal sinus is usually not well developed until the tenth year of life, it is during the adolescent years that frontal sinusitis first occurs. Infection of this or the other sinuses may be acute or chronic. Predisposing factors include allergy, obstruction (as with a deviated septum), or environmental pollution.

Acute Purulent Sinusitis. Symptoms appear within 5 days of acute rhinitis and include fever, headache, localized pain, and occasionally swelling. The location of the headache may assist in pinpointing the involved sinus, along the distribution of the trigeminal nerve in posterior ethmoid sinusitis, in the suboccipital area in sphenoidal sinusitis and over the eyes and temples in anterior ethmoid sinusitis.

Headaches

The differential diagnosis of a headache in the adolescent includes migraine, cluster headaches, sinusitis, increased intracranial pressure (secondary to either a neoplasm or pseudotumor cerebri), and infections (such as encephalitis or meningitis) (see p. 116).

Eyes

Visual Disturbances. *Myopia.* Nearsightedness often results from the elongation of the globe during the pubertal growth spurt in genetically predisposed individuals.

Blurred or Double Vision. This may occur secondary to failure of alignment of the visual axes as a result of ocular muscular weakness (such as multiple sclerosis or myasthenia gravis), nerve palsy, proptosis, an orbital mass, or increased intracranial pressure.

Decreased Visual Acuity and/or Blindness. Peripheral visual loss suggests progressive retinal degeneration (see below). Tunnel vision, particularly if of sudden onset, may be a symptom of a conversion reaction, although a complete ophthalmologic examination is indicated to rule out other causes. Night blindness is commonly caused by vitamin A deficiency, but progressive retinal degeneration should also be considered. This rare condition may occur in Laurence-Moon-Biedl, in Stargardt disease, and in Best vitelliform degeneration. Rapid onset of night blindness suggests infection (such as gonorrhea or chlamydia), hypertensive encephalopathy, toxins, or trauma. Gradual loss of vision is more compatible with progressive retinal degeneration, cataracts, vasculitides, or malignancies such as leukemia, glioma, or craniopharyngioma. Retinal detachment, itself secondary to trauma, hypertension, uveitis, or leukemia, may cause gradual or rapid loss of vision or blurring, often accompanied by flashes of light and/or showers of floaters.

Hysterical blindness may often be distinguished from that of organic etiology by the preservation of pupillary constriction upon light exposure in the former.

Pain. Pain in the eye may be caused by increased intraocular pressure (glaucoma) or conjunctivitis. Conjunctivitis is typically associated with a discharge, often with itching (if allergic), tearing, and conjunctival hyperemia and/or edema.

Discharge. A purulent discharge suggests bacterial infection (for example, staphylococci, pneumococci, streptococci, gonococci, chlamydia). A watery discharge is more typical of a viral or allergic cause of the conjunctivitis.

Nose

Smell. *Anosmia.* Inability to smell is a characteristic finding in the syndrome of hypogonadotrophic hypogonadism (Kallman syndrome). A more common cause, however, is chronic rhinitis.

Abnormal Smell. The experience of smelling something bizarre or something no one else can smell suggests the possibility of temporal lobe epilepsy, tumor, or toxic or other psychosis.

Nosebleeds. Childhood nosebleeds have a tendency to decrease in frequency and severity after puberty. The exception to this observation is that menarche may be associated with the spontaneous onset of epistaxis. As in younger children, the most common cause of epistaxis in the adolescent is trauma caused by sports injury, "horsing around," or picking at the nose. Sinusitis, allergic rhinitis, forceful coughing, polyps, or cocaine abuse may also predispose to nosebleeds. Profuse bleeding from both nostrils that is difficult to control suggests the possibility of an acquired coagulopathy (secondary to thrombocytopenia) or hypertension in the adolescent, in contrast to the differential diagnosis of epistaxis in childhood, which, includes congenital vascular anomalies.

Discharge. The appearance of the discharge provides clues as to its etiology:

Clear. Allergies (usually associated with itching of eyes, persistent sneezing, pale mucosa); viral infections (most commonly due to rhinoviruses and coronaviruses (erythematous mucosa).

Bloody. Foreign body; chronic purulent discharge (see below).

Purulent. Acute respiratory infections (particularly those caused by bacteria) and chronic conditions such as sinusitis, polyps, cystic fibrosis, dysmotile cilia, or foreign body.

Face

Parotid Swelling. Mumps has become much less common than previously as a result of immunization. Among older adolescents, however, it is still possible to see some cases. Parotid swelling without fever or tenderness may be a sign of bulimia (see pp. 138–139). Although it is not certain whether this finding is caused by the large carbohydrate load consumed during a binge, or is secondary to vomiting, it may be seen in those who induce vomiting, whether normal or overweight (bulimics) or malnourished (bulimiarexics).

Patients with pediatric acquired immunodeficiency syndrome (PAIDS) who have acquired the disease perinatally have chronic parotid swelling that appears to persist for years. It is, however, too soon to know whether this finding will persist into adolescence or if adolescents who acquire the infection may eventually develop this finding.

The Ear

Pain (Otalgia). Ear pain may result from otitis media, bullous myringitis, or otitis externa. In otitis externa, pain is increased by movement of the pinna and/or pressure on the tragus. Pathology elsewhere may be misperceived as being in the ear, such as in arthritis of the temporomandibular joint, tooth abscess, tonsillitis or peritonsillar abscess. When pain is associated with hearing loss and discharge, an eosinophilic granuloma may rarely be the cause.

Discharge. *Purulent.* Purulent discharge suggests either otitis externa or a perforated tympanic membrane secondary to otitis media.

Bloody. The most common cause of a bloody discharge is trauma secondary to sudden external compression (a slap) or penetration by a foreign object. Less often, if may be caused by neoplasm (such as a rhabdomyosarcoma) of the middle ear or chronic inflammation.

Clear. Serous otitis media with an effusion that drains through a perforated tympanic membrane will produce a clear discharge. Head trauma, resulting in a defect in the external auditory canal or tympanic membrane, may cause leakage of cerebrospinal fluid through the ear.

Hearing Loss. Chronic infection of the external or middle ear can cause conductive hearing loss, whereas sensorineural loss is likely to result from inner ear or retrocochlear disease or from acoustic trauma. Acoustic trauma in adolescents most commonly results from exposure to rock music, fireworks, or gunfire.

Vertigo. Most adolescents with vertigo describe it as the sensation of spinning often associated with nausea. Causes of vertigo include Menière disease, labyrinthitis, disease of the eustachian tube–middle ear, disease of the central nervous system (such as migraine), or formation of a perilymphatic fistula between the inner and middle ears. The latter is typically caused by sudden barotrauma (for example, secondary to extreme physical exertion, scuba diving, or playing a wind instrument) or a cholesteatoma.

Tinnitus. Disease of the eustachian tube–middle ear or ingestion of high doses of aspirin may cause "ringing" in the ears.

Mouth

Teeth. Pubertal development is reflected in the pattern of eruption of teeth. The teeth may be affected by caries at this age or by hydrochloric acid in those who vomit repeatedly. Severe generalized tooth pain may be the first sign of leukemia that is infiltrating the jaw.

Bad Breath. Teenagers are typically self-conscious and often concerned about the way they smell. Accordingly, the health professional may be consulted because of a complaint of bad breath. Most often the concern is unsupported by examination, but a complaint of bad breath or difficulty tasting may suggest zinc deficiency or a purulent exudate on the tonsils or pharynx.

Pain. Pain in the mouth is usually caused by an ulcerated lesion (herpes type I infection), aphthous ulcers, and, less commonly in this age group, gingival stomatitis. Throat pain is most severe in pharyngitis caused by beta-hemolytic streptococci, Epstein-Barr virus (infectious mononucleosis), or a retropharyngeal abscess. The latter may be so severe as to prevent normal swallowing, resulting in drooling. When these symptoms are accompanied by difficulty in breathing, or stridor, or both, it should be considered an emergency situation because of the possibility of epiglottitis (often caused in this age group by *Hemophilus influenzae*). With the resurgence of measles in the adolescent age group, Koplik spots (sand-like particles near the parotid duct on the buccal mucosa) may be found.

Tongue

The tongue often reflects systemic illness, vitamin deficiency, or antibiotic therapy. It may become sore, erythematous and strawberry-like in toxic shock syndrome or scarlet fever. A sore tongue is one of many symptoms of niacin deficiency. Patients on continuous antibiotic therapy occasionally develop a black hairy tongue (lingua negra). In this condition, the filiform papillae elongate in a triangular area in front of the V formed by circumvallate papillae. The so-called geographic tongue (prominent red and edematous papillae) has smooth red patches of desquamated filiform papillae, is usually asymptomatic, and is of unknown etiology.

Neck

A complaint of neck pain suggests the possibility of a strain of the sternocleidomastoid muscle, lymphadenopathy, thyroiditis, mass lesion, or meningitis, depending on the precise location of the pain as well as the presence or absence of other signs and symptoms.

RESPIRATORY SYSTEM

A **cough** in the adolescent may be acute or chronic, each suggesting different diagnostic possibilities. An acute cough may be due to a variety of viral etiologies, or to pneumococcal or chlamydial disease. The possibility of asthma should be considered. A chronic cough may be caused by tuberculosis or smoking. Rarely, in certain parts of the western U.S., an acute or chronic cough, accompanied by fever, may be due to coccidioidomycosis.

Respiratory depression may be a complication of drug overdose from opiates, barbiturates, or alcohol (see pp. 160–163).

Respiratory distress may occur secondary to asthma, pneumothorax, or aspiration of a foreign body.

Chest pain may accompany pneumonia, pleuritis, trauma to a rib, osteochondritis, pericarditis, pulmonary embolus, or pneumothorax (see pp. 119–124).

Breasts

A history of the timing of breast development in females should be ascertained to determine whether puberty is progressing normally. In males, the presence of enlarged or painful breasts suggests gynecomastia, which occurs in one-third to one-half of normal males, usually at SMR 3. The mass may be a discrete disk beneath the nipple and should not be mistaken for a tumor, a rare event in males of this age group. Pain in the breast of an adolescent female is most likely hormonally determined, being most severe premenstrually. Another common cause of breast pain is a cyst. The finding of a mass on self-inspection is most often a cyst or fibroadenoma, with tumors occurring rarely (cystosarcoma phylloides being more common than carcinoma in this age group).

A nipple discharge suggests the possibility of elevated prolactin levels (owing to pituitary adenoma, ingestion of certain medications such as phenothiazines or methyldopa, hypothyroidism), or, rarely, to infection or ductal neoplasm. Description of the color and consistency of the discharge may be helpful in distinguishing among these possibilities.

Heart

Chest Pain. In an otherwise healthy adolescent, chest pain is rarely of cardiac origin (see pp. 119–124). Myocardial ischemia may rarely occur, however, in an individual with aberrant left coronary artery, which may result in sudden death, usually on the athletic playing field.

Palpitations. Palpitations in this age group are most often due to premature ventricular contractions (PVCs), which typically result from ingestion of large amounts of caffeine. Other potentially more serious arrhythmias may cause palpitations and an ECG is warranted when the complaint is encountered. Holter monitoring may be necessary if the palpitations are intermittent. Dizziness may be of cardiac origin and may suggest postural hypotension, arrhythmia, prolonged QTc, or hypertrophic subaortic stenosis (the last is another cause of sudden death during athletic participation in a healthy-appearing adolescent). Patients with anorexia nervosa may die as the result of a ventricular arrhythmia, often presaged by prolongation of the QTc to more than 0.44 sec.

GASTROINTESTINAL SYSTEM

Vomiting

Acute onset of vomiting accompanied by fever suggests a number of possibilities in the adolescent: viral gastroenteritis, hepatitis, appendicitis, meningitis, encephalitis, poisoning with certain toxins (such as mushrooms), toxic shock syndrome, or salpingitis. Hepatitis in the adolescent is often secondary to infectious mononucleosis, although hepatitis A or B or non-A, non-B hepatitis may also occur. Acute vomiting in the afebrile adolescent may be a sign of alcohol intoxication, and is typically associated with slurred speech, unsteady gait, or coma; vomiting may be life-threatening when it causes aspiration. Pancreatitits as a cause of acute vomiting is rare in this age group, but may be a complication of chronic alcohol abuse. When vomiting is accompanied by headache and/or visual disturbance, increased intracranial pressure (such as may result from a tumor or pseudotumor cerebri) should be suspected, as should meningitis or encephalitis. The possibility of pregnancy should always be considered in the female adolescent with vomiting. Recurrent vomiting is suggestive of achalasia or Crohn disease, or may be self-induced, as in bulimia or anorexia nervosa.

Diarrhea

Acute gastroenteritis, caused by enteroviruses, is probably the most common cause of diarrhea. Nevertheless, hepatitis, dysentery from yersinia, campylobacter, giardia, and amebic infections should also be considered and ruled out by appropriate cultures. The sudden onset of profuse, watery diarrhea following myalgias, fever, and hypotension suggests the possibility of the early onset of toxic shock syndrome from the exotoxin of Staph 29/52. Although this problem is more common in females using tampons during menses, it may also occur following an abscess in either sex or the use of an intravaginal contraceptive device. Chronic diarrhea may be a symptom of inflammatory bowel disease, such as Crohn disease or ulcerative colitis, in which patients may have the full-blown disease—evidence of delay in pubertal development, weight loss or failure to gain age-appropriate weight, fever, blood in stools, anemia, and elevated erythrocyte sedimentation rate—or they may have an isolated sign or symptom. Lactose intolerance (secondary to deficiency of lactase in the intestinal villi) often has its onset during adolescence and is most common in Black and Oriental males, although it may occur in females and youngsters of any ethnic background. The typical history is that of bloating and diarrhea following ingestion of dairy products. The use of laxatives in an attempt to lose weight should also be considered in the differential diagnosis of chronic diarrhea in adolescents of either sex. Although it is less common during adolescence than at earlier ages, encopresis may be responsible for chronic overflow diarrhea.

Rectal Pain

The most common cause of rectal pain, particularly that associated with defecation, is a mucosal tear. Hemorrhoids are a rarer cause but start to be seen during adolescence. Tenesmus, a spasmodic pain, may be a symptom of gonococcal proctitis, in which there may be a purulent discharge from the anus. A lesion such as that caused by herpes type II or condyloma accuminata may also be associated with painful defecation. A perineal fistula, caused by Crohn disease or, less commonly, by lymphogranuloma venereum, may also cause pain in this general region. Pain in the absence of physical findings may be a symptom of rectal intercourse.

Jaundice

Onset of jaundice during adolescence may be caused by hepatitis, hemolysis, cholestasis, or obstruction. The differential diagnosis of hepatitis includes infectious mononucleosis (the most common etiology), hepatitis A, B, or non-A, non-B hepatitis. Hemolysis is rare at this age, except in patients who are chronically ill as, for example, those with sickle cell anemia, thalassemia, or G-6-PD deficiency. The acute onset of hemolysis may be secondary to exposure to a toxin such as warfarin. Cholestasis in the adolescent female is typically caused by either pregnancy or use of oral contraceptives, secondary to estrogens in both cases. Obstruction to bile flow may be caused by gallstones or by cirrhosis or fibrosis of the liver, the latter two being quite rare in the adolescent age group. Gallstones are rare before adolescence but increase in frequency, particularly in females, thereafter. Gallstone formation may result from hemolytic anemia, urinary tract infections, or obesity.

GENITOURINARY SYSTEM

Dysuria

The differential diagnosis of pain on urination in the adolescent includes cystitis and urethritis in both sexes, prostatitis in males, and vaginitis in females. Cystitis may be caused by viruses or bacteria. The pain is typically spasmodic and worsens at the completion of urination. Urethritis is most commonly caused by chlamydia or gonococcus. Rarely, mycoplasma species may be responsible. The syndrome is well described in males, in whom the former typically causes a clear, mucoid discharge, in contrast to that produced by gonococcus, which is yellow and thicker. Urethritis may be a part of the symptom complex of Reiter syndrome, which also includes arthritis and conjunctivitis.

Prostatitis

Prostatitis in the adolescent is almost always caused by gonococcus, which produces painful swelling of the gland resulting in painful urination.

Vaginal or Cervical Discharge (Table 16)

A clear, mucoid discharge that varies in amount at different points in the menstrual cycle, being most copious at mid-cycle, or that appears in the premenarcheal, virginal adolescent without a history of fever, pruritus, or dysuria is typical of a "physiologic" discharge. The appropriate response to such a history is education and reassurance. On the other hand, a foul-smelling yellow, brown, or green discharge accompanied by dysuria, pruritus, dyspareunia, and/or fever indicates a pathologic condition and mandates that a wet preparation and appropriate cultures be performed. If these procedures fail to elucidate the causative organism, *Gardnerella vaginalis* should be ruled out by appropriate cultures. The finding of clue cells on the wet preparation may be suggestive, as will a "fishy" odor when potassium hydroxide is added to a wet preparation. A white cheesy discharge with an acrid, sweet odor, pruritus, and dysuria constitute the usual history in a monilial infection. Rarely, pinworms and varicella may produce a discharge, the former being associated with pruritus, particularly at night, and the latter with vesicular lesions in the vaginal mucosa and elsewhere. The finding of a purulent discharge in an adolescent with a generalized rash, including palms and soles, who is febrile and has a history of dizziness and diarrhea should be regarded as an emergency, as it is likely to be an instance of toxic shock syndrome. Immediate attention will need to be given to cardiovascular support and institution of antistaphylococcal beta-lactamase resistant antibiotics.

Hematuria

In addition to diseases considered in children with this symptom, such as glomerulonephritis, hemolytic-uremic syndrome, and Henoch-Schönlein purpura, adolescents with hematuria may be experiencing the after-effects of strenuous endurance exercise, have cystitis, or, uncommonly a kidney stone.

Hematospermia

Trichomonas infection has been reported to cause this symptom.

TABLE 16. The Differential Diagnosis and Treatment of Vaginal Discharge in the Adolescent

			Bacterial						
	Viral *(Herpes Type 2)*	Chlamydia	*Gonococcus*	*Streptococcus*	Protozoan (Trichomonas)	Fungal (Candida)	Metazoan (Pinworms)	Physiologic	Irritant or Foreign Body
Appearance of discharge	Purulent	Purulent and frothy/ clear	Purulent	Purulent	Purulent or frothy	Cheesy	Clear to purulent	Clear mucoid	Purulent
Local signs and symptoms	Vesicles or none	Dysuria, dyspareunia or none	Pruritus Dysuria, dyspareunia or none	Pruritus Dysuria or none	Pruritus Dysuria or none	Pruritus Dysuria	Pruritus	None	Dysuria
Systemic signs (fever)	Occasionally	Present or absent	Present with acute salpingitis	None	None	None	None	None	None
Wet preparation	Polymorphonuclear leukocytes	Polymorphonuclear leukocytes	Polymorphonuclear leukocytes	Polymorphonuclear leukocytes	Polymorphonuclear leukocytes; Trichomonas	Epithelial cells	Polymorphonuclear leukocytes	Epithelial cells	Polymorphonuclear leukocytes
Culture	Viral media	Chlamydia growth media	Lester-Martin media in CO_2	Blood agar		Nickerson media	(Scotch tape preparation)		(Mixed flora staphylococci)
Treatment	Acyclovir 400 mg tid × 10 days	Doxycycline 100 mg bid × 7 days or erythromycin 500 mg qid × 7 days	Ceftriaxone 125–250 mg/m *or* amoxicillin 3 gm PO × 1; probenecid 1 gm PO *or* spectinomycin 2 gm IM*	Benzathine penicillin 1.2 million units IM	Metronidazole 2.0 gm PO once	Butaconazole cream HS × 3	Mebendazole 100 mg PO once	Reassurance	Removal
Treatment of contacts	None	Same	Same	None	Same	None			

*If allergic to penicillin or if organism is penicillin-resistant.

Menometrorrhagia

Menometrorrhagia describes excessive and frequent menstrual bleeding (see pp. 101–103 and Table 25). In determining its etiology, it is useful to consider whether the bleeding is painful or painless.

Causes of painful bleeding include those related to pregnancy (such as threatened abortion or ectopic pregnancy), salpingitis, or trauma. Traumatic causes include sports injury, such as water skiing, or intercourse, either forced (rape) or consensual (with the first intercourse). Sensitive interviewing skills and an appropriately private setting are necessary to obtain an accurate history under these circumstances.

The category of painless menometrorrhagia includes coagulopathies, either congenital or acquired. Although von Willebrand disease is a congenital condition, it may not present a problem until the time of menarche, when it may cause exsanguinating hemorrhage. Acquired coagulopathies include those that affect platelet function or number. Sensitivity to the acetyl moiety of acetylsalicylic acid (ASA) is manifested by problems of platelet adhesiveness, often causing excessive menstrual bleeding within 20 days of ingestion of a prescribed amount of the drug. Thrombocytopenia may also cause this symptom, and in this age group may result from leukemia, aplastic anemia, or idiopathic thrombocytopenic purpura (ITP).

Painless, excessive vaginal bleeding may result from hypothyroidism, and occasionally is the first symptom of this condition. Erratic use of oral contraceptives may cause excessive withdrawal or breakthrough bleeding. Neoplasms such as leiomyomata or endometrial carcinoma, which are the greatest concern when menometrorrhagia occurs in an adult woman, are exceedingly rare in adolescents, making a curettage procedure inappropriate for most in this age group. The primary gynecologic neoplasm in the adolescent with vaginal bleeding—adenocarcinoma—is rare and typically presents with vaginal spotting rather than excessive menstrual flow. Adenocarcinoma of the vagina occurs during puberty in those who were exposed in utero to diethylstilbestrol (DES) (primarily prior to 1970). The most common cause of menometrorrhagia in the adolescent has been given the name dysfunctional uterine bleeding (DUB). This condition results from anovulatory cycles in the year to 18 months following menarche. Consequently, estrogen is unopposed by progesterone, causing the buildup and consequent erratic shedding of proliferative endometrium.

Dysmenorrhea

Painful menses is a common problem among adolescent females, with one-third reporting this symptom (see also pp. 98–101, Table 24 and Fig. 11). Dysmenorrhea is categorized as primary or secondary. Primary dysmenorrhea is caused by excess production of prostaglandins F2α and E2 by the endometrium. Contrary to popular belief, this form of dysmenorrhea may occur from the time of menarche, although approximately half of patients do not experience pain until a year to 18 months later, presumably associated with the onset of regularly ovulatory cycles. Excess prostaglandin production is often responsible for the nausea, vomiting, and diarrhea that may accompany menstrual cramps.

Primary dysmenorrhea has been further subclassified as congestive or spasmodic, the former describing the combination of lower abdominal dull, aching pain associated with irritability, fatigue, constipation, and weight gain. This symptom complex may begin 2–4 days prior to and is relieved by menstrual onset. This form of dysmenorrhea may be part of the syndrome of premenstrual distress (PMS), related to decreases in levels of estrogens at this phase of the menstrual cycle, and is less common in adolescents than is the spasmodic variety. Spasmodic dysmenorrhea is the term used to describe sharper, labor-like lower abdominal pain that may radiate to the inner and anterior aspects of the thighs and lower back, often accompanied by vomiting, nausea, and diarrhea and lasting approximately 48 hours after onset of menses. This form of dysmenorrhea is related to increased levels of prostaglandins, as well as sensitization of the myometrium to their effects by progesterone produced by the corpus luteum in the ovulating adolescent.

Secondary dysmenorrhea results from an underlying structural abnormality such as relative cervical stenosis or endometriosis. Although pelvic and rectovaginal examination may assist in differentiating between these two forms of dysmenorrhea, a therapeutic trial of prostaglandin inhibitors (such as sodium naproxen) or ovulation inhibitors (such as oral contraceptives) is usually more helpful diagnostically. When these therapeutic interventions fail to alleviate symptoms, laparoscopy may be helpful in identifying endometriosis.

Premenstrual syndrome, also referred to as the late luteal phase dysphoric disorder, consists of affective symptoms such as depression, anxiety, and anger associated with severe impairment of psychosocial functioning in the days prior to menses. This is less common among adolescents than is dysmenorrhea, and is thought to be related to decreased estrogen levels.

Amenorrhea

Amenorrhea, or absence of menses, may be primary or secondary (see also pp 103–114). Primary amenorrhea refers to absence of menarche, whereas secondary amenorrhea describes cessation of menses for at least 3 months in a previously menstruating individual. Primary amenorrhea may be diagnosed in a young girl who fails to have menarche by the age of 16 years, or who does not begin to menstruate by the time she is 1 year older than was her mother at the time of her menarche, who has a bone age of 14½ years, or who has not had onset of pubertal development (SMR 2) by the age of 11 years. The differential diagnosis of primary amenorrhea is quite long (see Table 26). A history of unprotected intercourse should prompt performance of a pregnancy test (beta-HCG) even with primary amenorrhea. A history of weight loss, resulting from starvation, self-induced purging, endurance athletics, or chronic illness should be sought as possible explanations for this finding. A history of monthly abdominal pain, with or without an enlarging abdominal mass, in a pubertally mature adolescent who has not yet experienced menarche suggests the possibility of an imperforate hymen or cervical stenosis.

Another common cause of amenorrhea (primary or secondary) in a pubertally mature individual is polycystic ovary syndrome, which may occur in this age group without associated obesity, acne, or hirsutism (features typically found in the older adult). Short stature, particularly if associated with wide-spaced nipples and web neck, points to the possibility of Turner syndrome or a variant thereof. A central nervous system tumor, such as a craniopharyngioma, may be responsible for pubertal delay, and symptoms of increased intracranial pressure should be sought. Symptoms of heat intolerance and thin hair, with or without weight loss, suggest possible hyperthyroidism, although amenorrhea may be the only symptom of this condition initially. Stress, either physical or emotional, is known to cause amenorrhea, as are many medications, both prescribed and illicit (see Table 30). Accordingly, review of systems should include inquiry about these issues. Secondary amenorrhea may occur as a result of the conditions that cause primary amenorrhea, with the only obvious exceptions being congenital and chromosomal anomalies.

Physical Examination of the Adolescent

VITAL SIGNS

Pulse

The normal pulse rate for the adolescent is between 60 and 80/min. Puberty is associated with an increase in pulse rate in the male only. Athletes, in excellent physical condition, may have pulse rates somewhat slower than this, but any patient with a pulse rate below 50/min should be evaluated further, as this is below that commonly associated with peak cardiovascular fitness. In adolescents, the most common other cause of a slow pulse is anorexia nervosa. In this condition, the pulse may fall as low as 22/min in our experience, although the usual range is between 40 and 50/min. There is an obvious danger associated with bradycardia below 45/min, so that a complete cardiac evaluation and close cardiac monitoring are indicated to be sure that the patient is not at risk for an arrhythmia and sudden death. When hypothermia is present along with bradycardia in the patient with anorexia nervosa, it is often useful to warm the patient to 36.2°C, as this is usually followed by an increase in heart rate. Other causes of slow pulse include a prolonged QT interval, atrioventricular (AV) block, sick sinus syndrome (bradycardia alternates with tachycardia), and myxedema.

A rapid heart rate in adolescents suggests the possibility of paroxysmal atrial tachycardia (PAT), hyperthyroidism, or effects of pharmacologic agents such as caffeine (found in chocolate, cola drinks, over-the-counter stimulants), cocaine, amphetamines, or marijuana. An irregular pulse in an adolescent is typically due to premature ventricular contractions (PVCs), which may occur spontaneously or occur secondary to sensitivity to caffeine.

Blood Pressure

Blood pressure normally increases during puberty, particularly in males. Half of those destined to have essential hypertension as adults will manifest occasional (labile hypertension) or persistent elevations of blood pressure during adolescence. Accordingly, it is important to use age-specific reference standards for normal range of blood pressure for adolescents (Table 17). As at other ages, the proper technique for obtaining blood pressure should be used:

- Selection of proper cuff size (the largest cuff that will fit snugly, the bladder completely encircling the arm without overlapping).
- Proper positioning of the patient (a comfortable sitting position with the right arm fully exposed and extended, resting with support at the level of the heart).
- Application of the cuff with its lower edge above the antecubital fossa and placement of the diaphragm over the brachial artery.
- Proper inflation and deflation: rapid inflation to approximately 30 mm Hg above the point of disappearance of the radial pulse, followed by deflation at a rate of about 3 mm Hg/sec. The systolic blood pressure is that at which a clear tapping sound begins. When the tap changes to a low-pitched, muffled, softer sound, that is the diastolic blood pressure.

Temperature

Body temperature in the adolescent is the same as that in younger children and older adults, although the causes of lowered or increased temperature may be somewhat different. For example, the most common cause of hypothermia in the adolescent female is anorexia nervosa. In this condition, among the most malnourished, temperature during the night may fall as low as 33°C (93.2°F). Overdose of narcotics or alcohol may also cause hypothermia.

Increased body temperature may result from infection, neoplasm, hyperthyroidism, or transiently from rigorous-endurance aerobic exercise, or may be factitious. Illicit or prescribed drugs, such as amphetamines, hallucinogens, and anticholinergics may elevate body temperature. Measurement of basal body temperature may be useful in evaluating or reassuring a young female patient concerned about her ability to conceive.

HEIGHT

Height should be measured in the standing individual and the result plotted on a height velocity curve (Fig. 9) in order to evaluate whether the growth spurt has begun and its pattern. Failure to commence the height

TABLE 17. Correlation Between Blood Pressure and Stage of Pubertal Maturation

MALES

Age	Systolic Blood Pressure	Stage of Pubic Hair Development	Diastolic Blood Pressure	Stage of Pubic Hair Development
10	110 ± 9.0	0.26	59 ± 9.6	0.17
11	109 ± 9.5	0.24	59 ± 10.1	0.14
12	114 ± 10.1	0.25	58 ± 11.2	0.16
13	113 ± 10.3	0.42*	55 ± 10.9	0.13
14	116 ± 10.6	0.24	58 ± 9.0	0.25

FEMALES

Age	Systolic Blood Pressure	Stage of Breast Development	Menarche	Diastolic Blood Pressure	Stage of Breast Development	Menarche
10	108 ± 9.3	0.00	—	63 ± 7.8	−0.2	—
11	110 ± 9.8	0.19	−0.45**	59 ± 7.4	−0.24	−0.14
12	113 ± 9.4	0.08	−0.14	58 ± 11.8	0.01	0.1
13	112 ± 10.0	0.19	0.11	59 ± 9.6	0.18	0.1
14	115 ± 7.2	−0.09	−0.41**	66 ± 9.8	−0.24	−0.06

Modified from Londe S, Johanson J, Kronemer NS, et al: Blood pressure and puberty. J Pediatr 87:896–900, 1975.
*P = <.01.
**P = <.05.

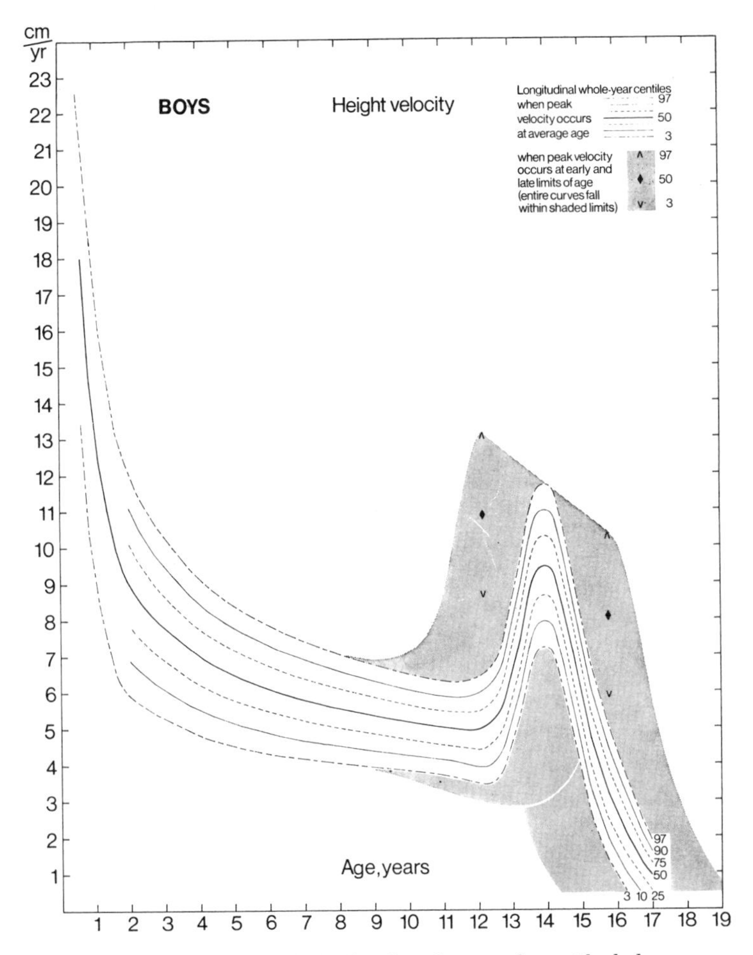

FIGURE 9. Longitudinal standards for height velocity in boys. Shaded areas represent total of hatched areas in upper and lower; it thus encloses all velocity curves within 3rd and 97th centile limits for age and for peak velocity. The 3rd, 50th, and 97th centiles for early- and late-maturing boys are indicated by arrowhead and diamond symbols. (From Tanner JM, Whitehouse RH, Takaishi M: Standards from birth to maturity for height, weight, height velocity, weight velocity: British children, 1965. Arch Dis Child 41:454–635, 1966, with permission.)

spurt in males by the age of 14 years (SMR 4) or in females by the age of 12 years (SMR 3) suggests the need for evaluation, unless the family history is similar.

WEIGHT

As for height, weight should be plotted on a velocity curve (Fig. 10). The peak of the weight velocity curve normally occurs approximately 6 months

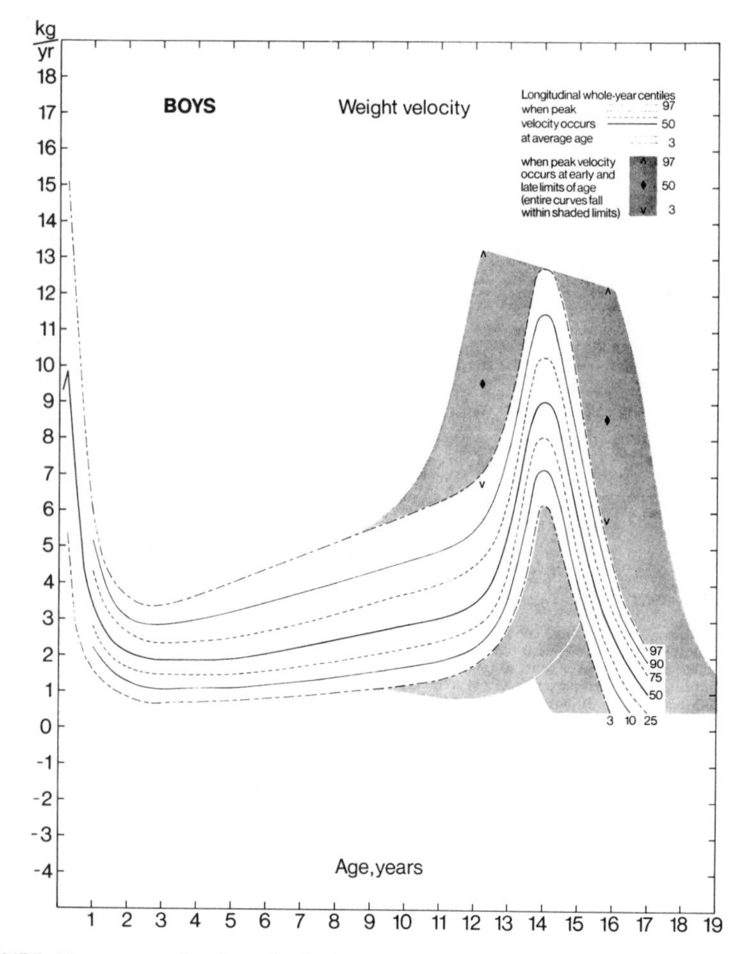

FIGURE 10. Longitudinal standards for weight velocity in boys. Shaded areas as in Figure 9. (From Tanner JM, Whitehouse RH, Takaishi M: Standards from birth to maturity for height, weight, height velocity, weight velocity: British children, 1965. Arch Dis Child 41:454–635, 1966, with permission.)

after that for height in females (approximately at SMR 3–4) and coincident with SMR 4 for males. The percentile for weight should correspond roughly to that for height. Body mass index (BMI) is commonly used for expressing weight in relationship to height (BMI = weight (kg)/height (cm)^2).

BODY FAT

During puberty, the increase in weight experienced by the female is almost entirely due to an increase in adipose tissue. From the childhood figure of 8% for both sexes, the percentage of the body that is fat increases to approximately 17% at SMR 4 and to 25% by completion of SMR 5 in females.

TABLE 18. Relationship of Skinfold Thickness to Percent Body Fat

Boys		Girls	
Skinfold Thickness (inches)	*Percent Body Fat*	*Skinfold Thickness (inches)*	*Percent Body Fat*
¼	5–9	¼	8–13
½	9–13	½	13–18
¾	13–18	¾	18–23
1	18–22	1	23–28
1¼	22–27	1¼	28–33

From Smith N, et al: Handbook for the Young Athlete. Palo Alto, CA, Bull Publishing Company, 1978, with permission.

The percentage of body fat decreases in males by the completion of puberty owing to the increase in muscle tissue at this time. Body fat measurement is an inexact science. Rough approximations may be made by measurement of skinfold thickness at different sites. A skinfold thickness of one inch corresponds to body fat percentage of 18–22% for boys and 23–28% for girls, and so forth (Table 18). The distribution of fat in the body also differs between the sexes, with more fat accumulating on the trunk in males, and more on both the trunk and extremities in females during puberty. Girls gain more subcutaneous fat in the lower segment of the trunk.

THE EYES

Paralysis of Accommodation

This condition may occur secondary to local instillation of anticholinergic drugs, with infections such as diphtheria, and with third nerve paralysis resulting from trauma, a vascular lesion, degenerative disease (such as multiple sclerosis), or a neoplasm. It may also be psychogenic in origin.

The Iris

Color change in the iris results from trauma, hemorrhage, glaucoma, inflammation (such as uveitis), or neoplasm. The appearance of nodules suggests neurofibromatosis, whereas infiltration occurs in leukemia.

The Pupil

Distortion and/or displacement of the pupil is a sign of tears or prolapse of the iris. Fixed or dilated pupils are found in drug overdose, in pinealoma, and in transtentorial herniation (Hutchinson pupil); the last is usually unilateral and often secondary to a subdural hematoma in this age group.

Mydriasis may result from use of drugs such as amphetamines or PCP. Pupils constricted by opiates or propoxyphene (Darvon) will dilate upon administration of naloxone (.01 mg/kg). Hysterical blindness may be differentiated from organic visual loss by the fact that the pupil will respond normally to a bright light in patients with hysterical blindness.

Homolateral miosis, associated with ptosis, enophthalmus, elevation of the lower lid, and decreased facial sweating, is found in oculosympathetic paresis (Horner syndrome), and may be caused by a mediastinal tumor or a lesion in the neck, midbrain, or orbit. The miotic pupil of Horner syndrome will not dilate following instillation with 1–2 drops of cocaine, whereas the normally miotic pupil will do so within 20–45 minutes.

Nystagmus

In adolescents, acquired nystagmus may be caused by pathology at the cerebellar, brainstem, or cerebral level, with the most common cause being barbiturate or alcohol abuse.

The Lid

Ptosis occurs in Horner syndrome as well as in neurofibromatosis with an upper lid neuroma, intracranial lesions that affect the third nerve, trauma, inflammation, or myasthenia gravis.

Retraction is most commonly seen in thyrotoxicosis, with staring (Dalrymple sign), decreased frequency of blinking (Stellwag sign), and lag of the upper lid on downward gaze (von Graefe sign).

Swelling of the lid can occur with a hordeolum (internal involves the meibomian glands; external, the glands of Zeis or Moll) or chalazion.

Pigmented Lesions. Dermal nevi first appear at puberty.

Sclerae. Icterus in the adolescent suggests hepatitis, hemolysis, or cholestatic jaundice. In this age group, the most common cause of hepatitis is infectious mononucleosis. Other infectious agents, such as hepatitis A and B and non-A, non-B should also be considered, especially if the patient is an intravenous drug user. Hemolysis may result from a hemoglobinopathy or red cell enzyme deficiency. Cholestatic jaundice may be caused by estrogens (either in oral contraceptives or as the result of pregnancy), or, more rarely in this age group, by cholelithiasis. The finding of subconjunctival hemorrhage may suggest increased vascular pressure, which commonly results from vomiting (possibly self-induced, as in bulimia, or secondary to excessive alcohol ingestion) or from weight-lifting, and requires rapid intervention by the physician.

The Conjunctivae

Injection may be caused transiently by use of marijuana or alcohol. In the acutely ill patient with fever and a rash, the possibility of toxic shock syndrome should be considered.

Hyperemia with Discharge. *Purulent Discharge.* Consider the possibility of infection with gonococcus, chlamydia, staphylococcus, pneumococcus, *H. influenzae*, or streptococcus. If arthralgias and urethritis are also present, a diagnosis of Reiter syndrome should also be entertained.

Watery Discharge. Watery discharge is seen in viral infections, as well as in allergic conditions, the latter being associated with intense itching, tearing, and conjunctival edema.

The Lens

Opacities may result from trauma, treatment with corticosteroids, metabolic disease such as Wilson disease (opacities are either subcapsular or radiating anterior capsular), or postpubertal diabetes mellitus (punctuate "snowflake" opacities in the subcapsular layers).

The Retina

Pigmentary Changes. Spots in the macula with a grayish foveal reflex is found in Stargardt disease, an autosomal recessive condition that does not become symptomatic until early adolescence. Yellow-orange pigment in the macula, resembling the yolk of an egg, is characteristic of Best vitelliform degeneration, an autosomal dominant condition that is typically discovered during adolescence.

Hemorrhages and Exudates. Flame-shaped hemorrhages and "cotton-wool patches" are characteristic findings in hypertensive retinopathy. The latter may also be found with nonspecific hemorrhages in severe anemias. White-centered hemorrhages with exudates may be found in leukemia. Hemorrhages with deep and waxy exudates are common in diabetic retinopathy, which increases in incidence after onset of puberty.

Disc Changes. Papilledema (blurred disc margins with hyperemia and absent venous pulses) is found in hypertensive retinopathy, severe anemias, or in increased intracranial pressure resulting from a tumor, such as a craniopharyngioma, or from pseudotumor cerebri, possibly secondary to large doses of steroids, tetracycline, or vitamin A taken for treatment of acne. A pale disc is seen in optic atrophy. Cupping of the disc, on the other hand, suggests increased intraocular pressure (glaucoma).

Vascular Changes. In hypertensive retinopathy, the vessels take on a silver or copper-wire appearance (secondary to thickening of the vessel wall), whereas diabetic retinopathy is associated with microaneurysms (appearing as tiny red dots) and venous dilatation.

Visual Fields

Homonymous hemianopsia (temporal field cut of one eye and contralateral nasal field cut) is found in lesions of the optic radiations. Bitemporal hemianopsia is associated with a lesion at the optic chiasm, most commonly craniopharyngioma. Superior quadrant anopsia may be found in patients with temporal lobe (psychomotor) epilepsy secondary to structural lesions.

THE EARS

The External Canal

Inflammation. When inflammation is present along with greasy scales, a diagnosis of seborrheic dermatitis is probable. Vesicles, edema, and weeping lesions suggest contact dermatitis caused by poison oak/ivy in this age group. Inflammation with a purulent discharge is typical of otitis externa (often, "swimmer's ear").

Mass Lesions. These are rare but when present suggest osteoma or fibrous dysplasia.

Vesicles. Vesicular eruptions on the posterior wall accompanied by facial paralysis are likely to be caused by herpes zoster (Ramsay Hunt syndrome). They also may occur in contact dermatitis.

The Tympanic Membrane

A hyperemic, opaque, bulging, poorly movable tympanic membrane is the classic finding in otitis media. A retracted, opaque, tympanic membrane or one with an air-fluid level or bubbles suggests otitis media with an effusion. Serous or hemorrhagic blebs on the membrane are characteristic of bullous myringitis. Perforations are caused by trauma: a "slap" injury typically produces linear or stellate perforation of the anterior portion of the pars tensa. Penetration with a foreign object may result in perforations anywhere on the membrane.

Examination of the ears, as well as audiometry and testing for conductive or sensorineural hearing loss, is warranted in the evaluation of the adolescent patient.

THE SINUSES

Sinusitis

Examination reveals localized and extreme tenderness over the affected sinus. Increased tenderness upon tapping of the upper molars suggests maxillary sinusitis. Tenderness in the distribution of the trigeminal nerve is associated with posterior ethmoid sinusitis. Careful examination of the nose for the site of purulent discharge will also assist in identifying the involved sinus. For example, when the pus is seen in the superior meatus, it suggests the possibility of sphenoid or posterior ethmoid sinus involvement, whereas pus in the middle meatus points to the frontal, maxillary, or anterior ethmoid sinus.

THE NOSE

Bleeding

Bleeding typically originates from Kesselbach plexus on the anterior septum, and may result from cocaine use, chronic irritation, or "picking." Polyps may cause bleeding. Examination of the trunk is indicated to observe other manifestations of a coagulopathy, such as petechiae or ecchymoses.

Discharge

Clear: Allergies (mucosa typically pale, eosinophils in the nasal smear); viral infection.

Bloody: Look for a foreign body (rare in the adolescent).

Purulent: May be from sinusitis, polyps, cystic fibrosis, dysmotile cilia, foreign body, or acute bacterial infection (polymorphonuclear leukocytes).

Septum

Perforation or erosion may result from sniffing of cocaine or heroin. Congenital syphilis may rarely cause perforation.

Polyps

The most common cause of nasal polyps in the pediatric age group is cystic fibrosis, with chronic allergies and asthma being more common causes when they present during adolescence.

THE MOUTH

Teeth

A number of features of dentition of the adolescent are noteworthy. Erosion of enamel, particularly on the posterior aspects, suggests the possibility of recurrent vomiting. During puberty, the second and third molars should erupt, so that examination of the teeth provides another clue about development. Adolescence is also the time of the second peak in dental caries. If caries is not treated, an abscess may intervene and cause lymphadenopathy of the anterior cervical chain. Tenderness in all the teeth of upper or lower jaw is seen in leukemias.

Pharynx

Puberty is associated with involution of lymphoid tissue, including the tonsils. Infection of the pharynx may be caused by beta-hemolytic streptococcus (group A) or gonococcus, as well as viral agents. The presence of tonsillar exudate is suggestive of infectious mononucleosis, streptococcal infection, or often both in this age group. Patients who induce vomiting by digital insertion may have lacerations of the pharynx and may lose their gag reflex after a few months of this behavior.

Palate

Petechiae on pale soft palate and/or uvula are seen in infectious mononucleosis (EBV). Petechiae in association with erythema and edema are compatible with a diagnosis of scarlet fever.

Buccal Mucosa

With measles now occurring most commonly in adolescents, the presence of Koplik spots should be sought in the febrile teenager, especially in the presence of a rash and photophobia. The chewing of smokeless tobacco may cause plaques in the mandibulo-mucobuccal fold. Herpes, type 1 or 2, may be responsible for vesicular lesions. Recurrent ulcers may be a manifestation of cyclic neutropenia.

Tongue

Worm-like movements of the tongue are manifestations of fibrillation, resulting from muscle denervation.

The finding of a black-brown triangular patch anterior to the V-shaped line of circumvallate papillae is referred to as "hairy tongue," and may be caused by chronic use of antibiotics. A white, coated tongue through which erythematous papillae project (white strawberry tongue) is an early manifestation of scarlet fever. This coating desquamates after a few days, leaving the papillae prominent (red strawberry tongue). The latter may also be seen in toxic shock syndrome.

THE NECK

Lymph Nodes

Because puberty is normally associated with involution of lymphoid tissue, the finding of enlarged lymph nodes in the teenager is usually indicative of a pathologic process. Common infectious causes of enlargement of suboccipital and posterior cervical nodes are Epstein-Barr virus (infectious mononucleosis) and rubella. As indicated above, enlargement of anterior cervical nodes may result from pharyngeal or dental infection. A caseating cervical node is seen in scrofula (tuberculosis), and is among the most common presentations of this infection in adolescents. Hodgkin and non-Hodgkin lymphomas make their appearance during adolescence, so that lymph node enlargement at any site should be carefully evaluated for this possibility. The finding of lymphadenopathy in an intravenous drug-using, sexually promiscuous, or hemophilic adolescent should raise concern about the possibility of HIV infection. Cat-scratch fever may be the explanation for lymphadenopathy in the febrile patient.

Torticollis may be spontaneous or result from a reaction to haloperidol-like medication or PCP.

Crepitus in the neck from rupture of an alveolar bleb with resultant pneumomediastinum and respiratory distress may occur spontaneously or as a result of self-induced vomiting.

Parotid Gland

Enlargement of the parotid in a febrile adolescent suggests mumps. Pediatric AIDS and bulimia may also cause enlargement.

Thyroid Gland

Enlargement of the thyroid gland suggests Hashimoto thyroiditis, a diagnosis confirmed by the finding of elevated levels of antithyroidal and antimicrosomal antibodies. In this condition, thyroid function tests may be normal or reflective of either hyperthyroidism or hypothyroidism. A goiter may be associated with either hyperthyroidism or hypothyroidism. Puberty is the time when malignancies of the thyroid gland first present, so that the finding of a nodule or asymmetric enlargement should be taken seriously and evaluated with a scan. Carcinoma of the thyroid is among the five most common cancers in females between the ages of 15 and 19 years.

THE CHEST

Completion of puberty is associated with expansion of the chest cavity and fusion of the sternoclavicular epiphysis in both sexes. Lung volume is also increased in males, with little appreciable change in females. Swelling at the sternoclavicular junction or at the point of attachment of any of the ribs to the sternum may occur with osteochondritis, a condition of unknown origin that is common in adolescents.

Cardiac Examination

By adolescence, most congenital cardiac conditions have been diagnosed. Aberrant left coronary artery syndrome and subaortic idiopathic hypertrophic stenosis may, however, defy diagnosis until they cause sudden death in an adolescent on the playing field. Mitral valve prolapse, suspected when there is a systolic click and confirmed by echocardiography, is being diagnosed with increasing frequency in adolescents, particularly females with other conditions such as scoliosis, panic attacks, and anorexia nervosa. Cardiac conditions that occur more commonly in adolescents than in younger children include premature ventricular contractions and prolonged QT syndrome. Extreme bradycardia (i.e., less than 45/min) in a thin adolescent should suggest anorexia nervosa and prompt the performance of an electrocardiogram to determine if potentially life-threatening prolongation of QTc is present.

Breasts

Males. Pathologic causes of gynecomastia are rare (see Table 12). Approximately one-third of adolescent males develop some breast tissue during puberty (idiopathic gynecomastia), typically at SMR 3. The mass is usually firm, subareolar, less than 4 cm in size, and may be tender. It may be bilateral or unilateral (80%). Its usual course is regression within 18 months of first appearance. A classification system for its evaluation is given in Table 19. Reassurance about its normality is the appropriate physician response. Only rarely is cosmetic surgery indicated.

Females. Breast development is one of the consistent secondary sex characteristics that appear during puberty. Asymmetric breast growth may be a cause of concern to a young woman. Reassurance is appropriate, particularly if puberty is still progressing. If the problem persists, wearing a padded bra may suffice. Rarely is reduction or augmentation mammoplasty indicated because of the morbidity associated with these operative procedures. Although it is customary to teach self-breast examination once breasts have developed, it is extremely uncommon for a breast malignancy to appear before the third decade. Breast masses in adolescent females are generally either cysts or fibroadenomas. A rare malignancy that is difficult to distinguish from a fibroadenoma on clinical grounds is cystosarcoma phyl-

TABLE 19. Classification of Gynecomastia

Type 1	Localized to subareolar area
Type 2	Generalized breast enlargement
Pseudogynecomastia	Increase in fatty tissue or hypertrophy of pectoral muscles, giving the appearance of breast enlargement*

loides. Increased pigmentation of the areola and enlargement of the surrounding Montgomery tubercles are found in pregnancy.

Nipple Discharge

A number of physiologic and pathologic conditions may be associated with a discharge from the nipple (Table 20). The most serious of these is a malignancy of the breast, which is exceedingly uncommon in adolescents. The most serious and common cause in adolescents of either sex is a prolactinoma. As indicated in the table, the appearance of the discharge can be helpful in determining its etiology. This process is facilitated by viewing a sample under the microscope and/or on a piece of gauze.

Appearance of the Discharge. *Milky.* A milky discharge is a spontaneous discharge from one or both nipples that has the consistency and color of skimmed milk and stains positive for fat globules. Although simple breast examination should not elicit a secretion, specific maneuvers such as squeezing the areola, or "stripping," a procedure in which pressure is applied to the breast from the base toward the nipple using both examining hands, will often accomplish this. A milky discharge so produced is referred to as galactorrhea when it occurs in the nonpuerperal individual, and is bilateral and persistent. It is often associated with amenorrhea. Prolactin levels are often found to be elevated (above 20 ng/ml), and prolactin inhibiting factor (PIF) low. Rarely, hypersensitivity of the end-organ (the breast) to normal levels of prolactin may be responsible for this finding. Causes of galactorrhea are listed in Table 21.

Grumous. A grumous discharge is a sticky substance that may appear bloody, but when viewed under the microscope or on a gauze pad will be found not to contain blood. This discharge is characteristic of ectasia of the duct (comedomastitis), a condition that causes redness, burning, itching, and swelling of the areola and nipple. The worm-like sensation appreciated when the areola is palpated has given rise to the term "varicocele" tumor of the

TABLE 20. Nipple Discharge

	Diagnosis			
Type	*Galactorrhea/ Fibrocystic Disease*	*Ectasia*	*Infection*	*Cancer*
Milky	XX			
Grumous		XX		
Purulent			XX	
Watery				X
Serous, serosanguinous, bloody	XX	X		XX

TABLE 21. Causes of Galactorrhea

- Endocrinopathies
- Intracranial neoplasms or trauma
  - Pituitary adenoma (prolactinoma [lactotrophinoma] or somatotroph)
  - Causing destruction of the PIF secreting center(s)
  - Causing section or compression of the pituitary stalk
- Trauma to thoracic wall (intercostal nerves T2–6)
  - Infection
  - Burn
  - Surgery
  - Atopic dermatitis
- Drugs (may cause galactorrhea in adolescents)
  - Hormones
    - Norethindrone (cyclical use)
    - Oral contraceptives (combination)—withdrawal
    - Estrogen—withdrawal
    - Methyltestosterone
    - Human chorionic gonadotropin
  - Psychoactive
    - Phenothiazines
    - Haloperidol
    - Benzodiazepines
    - Marijuana
    - Tricyclic antidepressants
    - Amphetamines
  - Antihypertensive
    - Reserpine
    - Spironolactone
    - Methyldopa
  - Other
    - Cimetidine
    - Isoniazid
- Hypothyroidism
- Chronic renal failure
- Bronchogenic or renal carcinoma
- Stress (emotional or physical)
- Anxiety
- Depression

breast. This condition is most common after the menopause but may occur in hypogonadal young women.

Purulent. The finding of pus cells in a nipple discharge is pathognomonic for infection. Mastitis occurs in the adolescent most commonly in association with the puerperium or lactation. A central abscess that may occur following trauma (such as a human bite) or in a diabetic adolescent may also cause a purulent discharge. Plasma cell mastitis is rare in the adolescent.

Watery. A watery discharge is uncommon and typically appears in association with an intraductal papilloma or cancer, the latter being rare in the adolescent patient.

Serous, Serosanguinous, or Bloody. The most common cause of this type of discharge is an intraductal papilloma, with fibrocystic disease being the next most common cause. Because the pathologic nature of the latter diagnosis is currently being questioned, it is probably appropriate to view such a discharge with suspicion, particularly because cancer is another cause, albeit less common, of this type of nipple discharge. Most patients reported have been in their fourth decade, but patients as young as 17 years have also been recognized with this type of discharge.

ABDOMEN

Skin

Increased pigmentation of the linea alba is associated with increased estrogenation, such as occurs in pregnancy. Extension of pubic hair up the linea alba occurs normally in some males who have passed SMR 5 (actually considered to be SMR 6 by some) but infrequently in females. In females, the condition may be familial (such as in those of Mediterranean descent) or associated with masculinization. Hair that is lighter and less coarse than mature pubic hair (lanugo) may be found on the abdomen, as well as the back and chest, in patients with anorexia nervosa.

Contour

A scaphoid abdomen is found in extreme weight loss such as occurs in anorexia nervosa. A protuberant abdomen may result from enlargement of any intra-abdominal organ, the most prominent of which may be an ovarian teratoma or pregnant uterus.

Tenderness

Tenderness to palpation of the abdomen is a common finding in patients of any age. Its significance is partly dependent upon the location at which pain is elicited and whether there is a history of pain prior to the examination. The presence of other symptoms and signs is also important. The combination of fever and abdominal tenderness should always be regarded as potentially serious.

Peritonitis. If tenderness is marked and localized or diffuse with rebound tenderness, abdominal guarding, or rigidity, peritonitis should be immediately suspected. First, the cause should be sought among illnesses more common among younger patients, such as ruptured appendicitis.

Among the possible causes of peritonitis, the following are most likely in adolescents:

- Appendicitis
- Inflammatory bowel disease with complications
- Gonococcal or chlamydial peritonitis in the sexually active female
- Ruptured ectopic pregnancy

Differential Diagnosis of Abdominal Tenderness

The cause of localized abdominal tenderness is usually suggested by the quadrant or region of the abdomen in which it appears; the history; the patient's sex; and the presence or absence of other signs or symptoms of disease.

Right Upper Quadrant Tenderness

RUQ tenderness in the adolescent suggests:
- Hepatitis
- Perihepatitis or cholelithiasis

Left Upper Quadrant Tenderness

Infectious Mononucleosis (EBV). Because the peak incidence of infectious mononucleosis occurs during adolescence, this diagnosis should always be considered in the adolescent with left upper quadrant tenderness due to an enlarged spleen. Palpation of the left upper quadrant in the febrile patient should be especially gentle to avoid rupture of an enlarged spleen.

Hodgkin Disease. An enlarged spleen may also be present in Hodgkin disease, although it is less likely to rupture in this disease.

Midepigastric Tenderness

- Ulcer disease
- Pancreatitis
- Repeated self-induced vomiting
- Hernia

Midline Tenderness Below the Umbilicus

- Infection of the bladder
- Endometritis
- A midline mass in an adolescent female associated with tenderness in this area suggests hematometrium or hematocolpos from an imperforate cervix or hymen, respectively.
- Pregnancy
- Abdominal muscle strain may also occur in young people who engage in weight-training, sit-ups, and other fitness programs or athletic activities.

Right Lower Quadrant Tenderness

- Appendicitis
- Inflammatory bowel disease
- Ectopic pregnancy
- Salpingitis
- Tubo-ovarian abscess

Left Lower Quadrant Tenderness

• The conditions listed under right lower quadrant except for appendicitis (unless situs inversus is present).

• Constipation is the commonest cause of left-sided abdominal tenderness in afebrile adolescent patients (especially in girls).

Emotional Causes of Abdominal Tenderness

School Avoidance. Diffuse abdominal tenderness in the absence of other signs and symptoms, especially when accompanied by excessive school absence, should suggest conversion reaction or school avoidance. Evaluation of psychosocial and organic causes of the symptom should be undertaken simultaneously.

Bulimia. Repeated vomiting in this disorder may also cause tenderness of the abdominal muscles.

Organomegaly

The finding of an enlarged **spleen** in the adolescent suggests either lymphoma, Hodgkin disease, hemoglobinopathy, or infectious mononucleosis. Palpation must be undertaken with extreme care when infectious mononucleosis is suspected, because rupture may result.

Enlargement of the **liver** in the adolescent may be associated with hepatitis, cirrhosis, fibrosis, or a tumor. The last three are rare unless there is preexisting metabolic or congenital disease.

Abdominal Masses

It is not unusual to palpate a large pulsating midline mass (which represents the aorta) in the area of the umbilicus in the thin adolescent female. A mass in the right lower quadrant may be secondary to a periappendiceal or pericecal abscess, complications of appendicitis or inflamatory bowel disease. A mass in either the right or left lower quadrants may represent an enlarged ovary (secondary to a cyst or tumor), tubo-ovarian abscess, ectopic pregnancy, or hydrosalpinx. As indicated above, a midline mass in the lower abdomen suggests intrauterine pregnancy or, if present in a pubertally mature female who has never menstruated, hematocolpos or hematometrium (a blood-filled vagina or uterus, respectively) in a patient with an imperforate hymen or cervical stenosis. The frequency of constipation in the otherwise normal, but busy, adolescent is a reminder that a left-sided abdominal mass may actually represent stool.

GENITALIA

Male

Inspection

As previously discussed, the character and distribution of pubic hair form the basis for assessment of pubertal development. Careful inspection of the pubic hair may reveal the presence of adherent eggs (lice) or folliculitis. The size of testes and stage of development of the penis will assist in evaluation of pubertal growth. A finding of urethral discharge suggests the possibility of a sexually transmitted disease or Reiter syndrome. A clear discharge is usually associated with chlamydia, whereas a purulent one is found with gonococcus.

The Penis

The descriptions of the conditions below are based on the presenting lesion. Not included in the discussion are diseases that occur after adolescence (such as squamous cell carcinoma or balanitis xerotica obliterans).

Papules. The size, distribution, and associated signs and symptoms can assist in identification of the cause of penile papules.

Tiny papules around the corona without associated signs or symptoms are typical "pearly penile papules." These shiny white papules, which are 1–3 mm in height, are distributed diffusely over the corona, without extention to the foreskin or glans. They may be more common on the anterior than posterior surface. They occur in postpubertal males and are rare before SMR 3. It is estimated that 20% of adult males have these benign lesions, which are of no consequence. Reassurance is the appropriate response.

A single tender papule on the shaft or glans may be the initial presentation of a number of sexually transmitted diseases:

Granuloma Inguinale. The papule rapidly becomes ulcerated. The ulcer is irregular in contour, covered with granulation tissue, and has raised margins. Characteristically, a new lesion develops at the periphery of the ulcer and, if untreated, an extensive mass of ulcerating and granulation tissue will envelop the genitals. Diagnosis is made by examination of a crushed smear of tissue stained with either Wright or Giemsa stain to reveal the Donovan body, a small bacillus with rounded ends that stain darker than the center.

Condyloma Acuminatum. The papule is wart-like in appearance (gray, rough, verrucous) and may become pedunculated. It grows beneath or on the prepuce, the glans, or coronal sulcus, or at the external meatus. The initially single papules may become confluent. They are caused by the papilloma virus (HPV), which has been shown to be premalignant. Diagnosis may be made by culture or electrophoretic techniques. Lesions in the asymptomatic partner of a patient with HPV infection may be made manifest by application of a mild solution of acetic acid, which renders the infected areas white.

Condyloma Latum. See p. 85.

Lichen Planus. The papule of lichen planus is purple, polygonal, and pruritic, and may be annular or dispersed in arrangement. The papules may be found on the glans or shaft of the penis and may be accompanied by lesions elsewhere on the body (extremities, buccal mucosa and/or tongue).

Macules. *Chancroid.* The initial lesion is a small macule on the prepuce posterior to the glans penis, which rapidly becomes pustular. The pustule ruptures, leaving a small ulceration with an erythematous base that resembles that of herpes progenitalis, both of which are extremely tender. As the ulcer grows, the edges become irregular and undermined, and the surface becomes covered by a grayish-yellow membrane. Phimosis may occur if the prepuce is redundant. Inguinal lymphadenopathy is commonly present and is initially tender, fixed, and matted, and soon becomes fluctuant. The lesion is caused by *Hemophilus ducreyi,* which is not commonly grown in most laboratories, so that the diagnosis is made on clinical grounds and on the response to sulfonamides or tetracycline. Herpes should be ruled out by appropriate cultures, as these lesions are very similar in appearance.

Gonorrhea. Disseminated gonococcemia may present a variety of lesions, including macules, which may be present anywhere on the body, even on the penis. The most common presentation of this sexually transmitted disease is with a urethral discharge.

Vesicles. *Herpes Progenitalis.* The typical primary lesion consists of large discrete vesicles on an erythematous base on the glans, prepuce, or shaft of the penis. They are extremely painful and pruritic. Their appearance is often heralded by hypersensitivity and severe pain along a sacral nerve distribution. The vesicle is fragile and may break, leaving a tender ulcerated lesion that often is difficult to differentiate clinically from that of chancroid. The lesions last for 2–4 weeks and may be accompanied by tender and enlarged inguinal lymph nodes. Recurrent herpes is characterized by the presence of clusters of minute vesicles on an erythematous base. These are also friable and, when broken, leave moist, tender superficial erosions. The usual duration of recurrent lesions is 7–10 days. Culture will reveal the virus, often suggested by the finding of multinucleated giant cells with a Wright stain of the contents of an intact vesicle (obtained by scraping the base of the vesicle with a No. 11 scalpel blade).

Contact Dermatitis. Grouped and often arranged linearly, these vesicles may result from direct contact with the irritant, or following sensitization, as with poison ivy or poison oak. These lesions are quite pruritic.

Painful Ulcers. As indicated above, the initial lesions of both chancroid and herpes progenitalis typically progress to painful ulcers on an erythematous base. The finding of multinucleated giant cells on Wright stain with confirmation by culture establishes a diagnosis of the latter, the former usually being diagnosed by response to therapy.

Painless Ulcers. *Primary Syphilis.* The lesion of primary syphilis is the chancre, which begins as a papule that later erodes into an indurated, painless ulcer. It is typically a single, sharply demarcated lesion on the shaft, occasionally is multiple, and rarely occurs on the glans. Inguinal lymphadenopathy is hard and nonsuppurating. Examination of scrapings from the base of the ulcer placed on a slide will reveal spirochetes when the fresh material is viewed through a darkfield condenser. Serologic tests are negative in 75% of patients at the time of initial appearance of these lesions, although they typically convert to positive within a few weeks.

Infectious Mononucleosis. There is but one case report of an adolescent with infectious mononucleosis who had a single, shallow, punched out lesion on his penis and a negative evaluation for other pathogens.

Scaly Lesions. *Psoriasis.* A sharply demarcated, bright red lesion with most and often crusted scales is characteristic of psoriasis. Scraping of the scales results in pinpoint bleeding sites. The lesions may occur on the penis alone or in conjunction with lesions elsewhere on the body.

Erythema. *Balanitis.* This nonspecific inflammation of the glans penis may be associated with poor hygiene and chronic irritation, and may occur in conjunction with inflammation of the prepuce.

Female

Inspection

The character and distribution of pubic hair form the basis for assessment of pubertal development. Inspection of pubic hair may also reveal the presence of adherent eggs (lice), lesions of scabies, or swelling of the hair follicle. Inspection of the external genitalia should include examination of the clitoris to ascertain whether or not it is enlarged, and of the hymen to determine if it is perforate. Determination of penetration by inspection of the hymen in the fully mature female is difficult and should not be undertaken. The presence of excoriations suggests infestation with scabies, pinworms, or *Candida albicans*. Raised papules may represent condyloma latum (the flat, smooth lesions of secondary syphilis) or condyloma acuminatum (gray, rough lesions caused by human papilloma virus).

Vesicles. Vesicles may be found with herpes simplex infection or, rarely in this age group, with varicella.

Fistulas. Fistulas in the perineum may be associated with Crohn disease or, less commonly, with lymphogranuloma venereum (LGV). A small, superficial lesion in the fourchette may be the primary lesion of LGV in which the more prominent finding is the presence of fluctuant inguinal lymphadenopathy.

Discharge. A vaginal discharge may be physiologic or infectious. The former may be distinguished by its color (white, mucoid), absence of foul odor, pruritus, or dysuria, as well as by the presence of epithelial cells with no other cell types on microscopic examination in a wet preparation (see Table 16).

In contrast, a discharge associated with infection is typically colored (either green, brown, or yellow, or white in the case of *Candida albicans*) and foul-smelling (except with candida), and is associated with pruritus or dysuria. A wet preparation that reveals polymorphonuclear leukocytes (in addition to normally present epithelial cells) usually indicates infection. The presence of trichomonads is diagnostic of trichomoniasis, but it is important to search for other sexually transmitted pathogens when one is found in the adolescent. Culture, using appropriate swabs (avoiding synthetics such as Dacron) and specific culture media and conditions, will permit specific diagnosis and appropriate antibiotic therapy (see Table 16).

Vaginal Mucosa. With advancing puberty, the vaginal mucosa becomes thicker, owing to increasing layers of cornified epithelium. These cells increase in glycogen content as well. As a result, the vaginal mucosa during puberty becomes more resistant to some pathogens (such as gonococcus) and more susceptible to others (such as candida and gardnerella). The mucosa should be inspected with the naked eye and good illumination, such as that provided by a fiberoptic vaginoscope inserted in a clear plastic speculum. A more careful view is provided by inspection of the mucosa through a colposcope, which allows for histologic examination of *in situ* and live cells. Such an examination is warranted when looking for vaginal adenosis or adenocarcinoma of the vagina in a patient with a history of prenatal exposure to diethylstilbestrol or for trichomoniasis or HPV. The colposcope is now being studied as an adjunct to examination following rape in children.

Cervix. Inspection of the cervix reveals additional useful information, such as the status of the cervical os (fishmouth configuration is usually associated with previous childbirth or abortion), erosion (the red, friable mucosa), and the presence of lesions such as a nontender chancre (syphilis).

Examination of the cervical mucosa through the colposcope may reveal a stippled appearance associated with trichomonas infection. It is difficult to diagnose cervical stenosis by inspection alone. The diagnosis is suspected from a history of scant menstrual flow and abdominal cramps. The position of the cervix has little clinical relevance. Current information suggests that there is no association between a retroverted uterus and dysmenorrhea, as was once taught. The position of the cervix is important in the process of fitting a diaphragm. If, for example, the cervix is reached before the posterior fornix when introducing an examining finger, one would prescribe an arched spring, rather than a flat spring, diaphragm. A low-lying cervix is more subject to trauma during intercourse; hence, there is a higher incidence of dyspareunia among women with this otherwise normal variant. A cyanotic cervix (Chadwick sign) is suggestive of pregnancy, although it is among the less reliable physical signs of pregnancy. The presence of a discharge or bleeding from the os should be noted and a sample taken if the origin is suspected of being anything other than physiologic. Absence of a cervix suggests a mullerian duct anomaly, which should be further evaluated initially with pelvic ultrasonography, followed by laparoscopy if the former is not diagnostic.

Palpation

Male

The presence of a scrotal mass (testicular tumor) or varicocele may be ascertained by palpation if this is not apparent by visual inspection alone.

Female

Palpation of the vaginal mucosa may reveal the presence of submucous or concealed lesions, such as condyloma (either acuminatum or latum), molluscum contagiosum, chancre, or a polyp (rare in this age group). Palpation of the cervix may reveal that it is soft, suggestive of pregnancy. Once establishing a level of discomfort (or, preferably, comfort), it is appropriate to rock the cervix gently from side to side. If this produces pain, it suggests that there is inflammation of the fallopian tubes or ligaments that anchor the cervix, the most likely cause of which is infection. Palpation of the rectovaginal septum and, if possible, of the suspensory ligaments, may reveal thickening and beading, suggestive of endometrial implants (endometriosis). These may be responsible for severe menstrual cramps (and other symptoms, determined by the location of the implants within the peritoneal cavity). Bimanual palpation should then proceed to include the uterus itself. An enlarged uterus is most commonly associated with intrauterine pregnancy in adolescents. Choriocarcinoma is rare and leiomyomata are even less common in adolescents. In the otherwise pubertally mature adolescent with primary amenorrhea, the finding of an enlarged uterus suggests hematocolpos caused by retained blood. Palpation of tenderness in the adenexa is compatible with salpingitis, particularly if it is accompanied by tenderness on cervical motion. Unilateral adenexa suggests an ectopic pregnancy, tubo-ovarian abscess, or hydrosalpinx, pyosalpinx, or ovarian cyst.

Guidelines for performance of a pelvic examination are found in Appendix 7. Discussion of the evaluation of the rape victim is found on pp. 150–154.

Rectal Examination

A rectal examination is not a part of the routine physical examination of the adolescent patient. It should be performed, however, when there is a history of rectal pain, penetration, bleeding, or discharge, or of urinary hesitancy in males. It is vital that a rectal examination be performed in any adolescent with an unexplained history of a limp or pain in the hip or knee. Inspection of the rectal area may reveal pathologic lesions such as a chancre, condylomata lata or acuminata, the primary lesion of lymphogranuloma venereum, a fistula (resulting from lymphogranuloma or Crohn disease), and, rarely in this age group, a hemorrhoid. A patulous anus suggests repeated anal intercourse. Excoriations in the area of the anus may occur when there are pinworms. In the male, a rectal examination will allow for palpation of the prostate gland to determine if it is enlarged. At this age, the finding of an enlarged prostate, especially when associated with tenderness, is suggestive of an infectious process such as gonorrhea.

THE SKIN

Inspection

The skin of the adolescent may be regarded as another of the secondary sex characteristics, as it is exquisitely sensitive to the hormonal changes of puberty. Increasing levels of androgens, derived from testicular secretions in males and from the adrenals in both sexes, are converted to dihydrotestosterone, which acts to stimulate growth of sebaceous follicles and its secretions (sebum). When sebum is broken down to component fatty acids by the bacteria normally present on the skin *(Corynebacterium acnes)*, irritation may result, causing the lesions of acne (see Fig. 4).

Acne

The lesions of acne consist of comedones (blackheads), papules, pustules, and cysts. The location and severity of the lesions provide the basis for acne classification, such as that devised by Pillsbury (see Table 13). Treatment of acne is often based on such classification systems. Grades 1 and 2 are usually treated topically (for example, topical retinoic acid, benzoyl peroxide, clindamycin, erythromycin), whereas systemic antibiotics (such as tetracycline) are typically reserved for pustular grades. Cis-retinoic acid (Accutane) may be prescribed for nonpregnant adolescents with cystic acne.

Striae

Striae are thin, depressed bands of atrophic skin that initially appear erythematous and eventually turn silvery. They occur in areas that have undergone rapid growth, most commonly the breasts and thighs. They may also result from pregnancy, Cushing disease, obesity, or corticosteroid therapy.

Tattoos

Adolescents acquire tattoos (typically self-administered or done by other amateurs) to signal membership in a particular peer or religious group, gang, or activity. Tattoos are usually on the upper extremities, often between fingers, or in the "snuff box." Tattoos may also be positioned so as to disguise needle tracks. To detect them, it is useful to apply a tourniquet above the level of the tattoo and observe its location along the course of a vein. The old-fashioned practice of tattooing the name of a loved one is uncommon among today's teenagers. The fact that adolescents' tattoos are often done by amateurs means that nonsterile techniques may cause infectious complications such as hepatitis B, HIV, or infectious mononucleosis.

Rashes

The significance of rashes in the perineal and genital areas is addressed on pp. 82–85. Rashes elsewhere on the body may be caused by a number of conditions, as follows:

Erythroderma. A rash with the appearance of a sunburn in an adolescent without a history of solar exposure suggests toxic shock syndrome (see Table 22 for criteria for this diagnosis). This potentially fatal condition caused by certain strains of *Staphylococcus aureus* (29/52) occurs in conjunction with tampon use, but may result from use of contraceptive diaphragm or sponge or as a complication of surgery, influenza, or abscess.

Urticaria. Hives occur at all ages, but the adolescent's predilection for experimenting with new and unfamiliar substances places him or her at increased risk for allergic reactions.

Papules and Pustules. Pruritic pustules, particularly between fingers and on the abdomen and buttocks, are typical findings in scabies.

Vesicles. A pruritic, vesicular eruption is seen on the skin in poison oak/ivy. A painful vesicular lesion on the lips or buccal mucosa suggests herpes I. Varicella is rare, but may occur among adolescents. Disseminated gonococcemia may also produce vesicles.

TABLE 22. Revised Case Definition of Toxic Shock Syndrome

Fever: temperature ≥ 38.9°C (102°F)
Rash: diffuse macular erythroderma
Desquamation 1 to 2 weeks after onset of illness, particularly of palms and soles
Hypotension: systolic blood pressure ≤ 90 mm Hg for adults or below fifth percentile by age for children below 16 years of age, orthostatic drop in diastolic blood pressure ≥ 15 mm Hg from lying to sitting, orthostatic syncope, or orthostatic dizziness
Multisystem involvement—three or more of the following:
- Gastrointestinal: vomiting or diarrhea at onset of illness
- Muscular: severe myalgia or creatine kinase level at least twice the upper limit of normal for laboratory
- Mucous membrane: vaginal, oropharyngeal, or conjunctival hyperemia
- Renal: blood urea nitrogen or creatinine at least twice the upper limit of normal for the laboratory, or urinary sediment with pyuria (≥ 5 leukocytes per high-power field) in the absence of urinary tract infection
- Hepatic: total bilirubin, SGOT*, SGPT† at least twice the upper limit of normal for laboratory
- Hematologic: platelets ≥ 100,000/mm^3
- Central nervous system: disorientation or alterations in consciousness without focal neurologic signs when fever and hypotension are absent

Negative results on the following tests, if obtained:
- Blood, throat, or cerebrospinal fluid cultures (blood culture may be positive for *Staphylococcus aureus*)
- Rise in titer to Rocky Mountain spotted fever, leptospirosis, or rubeola

From Centers for Disease Control: Criteria for defining a case of toxic shock syndrome. MMWR 29:441–445, 1980.
*SGOT denotes serum aspartate transaminase.
†SGPT denotes serum alanine transaminase.

Macular Erythema. Should this appear in the form of blotchy, irregular lesions on the fifth day of a febrile illness, first on the face, then behind the ears with spreading to the chest and abdomen, and, finally, on the extremities, rubeola (measles) is the most likely diagnosis. Adolescents now have the highest incidence of this viral disease.

A faint eruption of discrete, fine, erythematous macules in an adolescent with a low-grade fever, malaise, and possibly enlarged suboccipital and/or epitrochlear lymph nodes suggests rubella (German measles) or infectious mononucleosis, both of which are also now more common among adolescents than other age groups.

An erythematous macule or papule that progresses to a large annular lesion with central clearing (erythema chronicum migrans) is characteristic of Lyme disease.

Macular plaques that are pink to purple and vary in size from a few millimeters to several centimeters may occur in sensitive individuals who ingest laxatives containing phenolphthalein. Adolescents with bulimia are the group at risk for this practice. These persistent lesions are often accompanied by pruritus and burning, and may proceed to vesiculation and ulceration. Exacerbation may be associated with subsequent use.

Café-au-lait Spots. These flat, brown areas of discoloration are associated with neurofibromatosis (von Recklinghausen disease). The lesions are asymptomatic, but their significance rests in that they signal the possibility of tumors of the peripheral or central nervous system.

Papules. Flat-topped, erythematous over knuckles—consistent with dermatomyositis. Acneiform, erythematous around nose—consider tuberous sclerosis.

Hyperpigmentation. For hyperpigmentation at the knuckles, palmar creases, scrotum, linea alba—consider Addison disease. Hyperpigmentation at areola, linea alba—consistent with pregnancy. Hyperpigmentation and papillary hypertrophy at skinfolds that result in a velvety appearance—consider acanthosis nigricans.

Fungal Diseases. Scaly, pruritic, erythematous patches that spread, with central scaling and often vesicles, resulting in a ring-like lesion, are typical of fungal disease. These may occur in the groin or scalp. Depending on the location of the lesion, they are labeled tinea cruris (inguinal area), tinea capitis (scalp), or tinea corporis (body), and may be caused by one of two species of fungi, Microsporum or Trichophyton. The former fluoresces under a Wood lamp, whereas the latter does not. A more reliable diagnostic method is scraping the lesion with a scalpel and viewing the material (to which potassium hydroxide had been added) through the microscope.

Bruises

Ecchymoses suggest either trauma or a bleeding diathesis. Trauma may result from an accident or from abuse. The folk-medicine practice of "coin-rubbing" among Southeast Asians produces linear ecchymotic streaks along the back. Ecchymoses on the trunk are more suggestive of a coagulopathy than are those appearing on the extremities alone. Inquiry about excessive bleeding from cuts, toothbrushing, and menses is appropriate when evaluating a patient with unexplained bruises.

Needle Tracks

Injection of drugs into veins with needles "sterilized" by passage through a flame results in the intradermal deposition of minute amounts of charcoal that accumulate over time to produce a darkened line. The associated fibrosis and thickening of the vessel contribute to the formation of so-called needle tracks.

Fluorescence

Exposure of normal skin to ultraviolet (Wood) light in a darkened room results in an orange glow caused by sebum. A patient who is compliant with tetracycline therapy produces sebum that manifests a greenish fluorescence under these circumstances (a quick method for assessing compliance!). Skin infected with fungi from the Microsporum species (which causes tinea corporis, cruris, or capitis) fluoresces under Wood light, whereas that infected by the Trichophyton species does not.

ORTHOPEDIC EXAMINATION

Back

For scoliosis, the examination should be performed from behind the patient. Observe the relative heights of the iliac crests. Instruct the disrobed patient to bend forward 90° with his or her hands clasped in the midline, and observe the symmetry of the rib cage. If the rib cage is higher on one side than the other (a hump), it suggests a rotation with lateral curvature. The presence of an actual curvature should also be noted. A curvature of 30° or greater will be apparent upon inspection alone. The finding of a lateral curvature of the spine with rotation of the vertebrae indicates scoliosis. In the most common type of scoliosis—idiopathic scoliosis—the apex of the convexity of the curve is to the left in the thoracic region, and is termed left thoracic scoliosis. When the apex of the convexity of the curve is to the right in the lumbar region, it is referred to as right lumbar scoliosis.

The examination should also include the observation of the patient from the side. The finding of an anterior curvature of the spine constitutes **lordosis.** This is normal in the lumbar spine. A posterior curvature of the spine is called **kyphosis,** although this is considered to be normal when it occurs in the thorax.

Differential Diagnosis of Scoliosis

Idiopathic scoliosis appears usually in postpubertal females and is accentuated with growth. Pathologic causes of scoliosis are listed in Table 23 and include congenital anomalies and acquired defects. A right thoracic curve is more typical of pathologic causes.

Evaluation. In addition to the orthopedic examination, the finding of scoliosis requires a careful neurologic examination. X-rays should be obtained of the spine with the patient in a standing position, both anteroposterior and lateral. The number of convexity of curves is thus documented and the magnitude of the curves quantified, as treatment is determined by the latter.

No treatment is indicated for curvatures less than 20°. Those between 20° and 40° are treated with bracing in adolescents whose pubertal growth spurt has not been completed. Spinal fusion is generally recommended for thoracic curves greater than 60° because of the increased risk of pulmonary

TABLE 23. Differential Diagnosis of Scoliosis in the Adolescent

Idiopathic
Asymmetry of Musculature
Cerebral palsy
Muscular dystrophy
Poliomyelitis
Hemihypertrophy
Hemiatrophy
Defects of Spinal Cord/Vertebral Column
Hemivertebra
Marfan syndrome
Herniation of nucleus pulposus
Spinal cord tumor
Spinal cord abscess
Neurofibromatosis
Asymmetry of Leg Length
Pseudo-scoliosis

compromise in later life. With curves of between 40° and 60°, treatment decisions will be based on rate of progression and symptomatology.

Kyphosis may occur during adolescence, more commonly in boys, as a result of enchondral ossification of the anterior portion of the vertebral bodies, which arrests growth anteriorly (Scheuermann disease).

Osteoporosis. Decreased bone density has recently been documented in certain groups of adolescent women: those with primary or secondary amenorrhea associated with anorexia nervosa or those with inappropriately treated Turner syndrome. The long-term significance of this finding and implications for treatment are unclear at this time. It is disconcerting, however, as the peak of bone density (200 mg/ml) is normally reached by the 20th birthday, with a 1–2% decrease yearly thereafter in premenopausal women.

Low Back Pain

Low back pain in the adolescent is most commonly mechanical in origin, but neoplastic, infectious, or skeletal disease (e.g., Scheuermann kyphosis) must also be considered. Mechanical causes include exaggeration of lumbar lordosis, tight lumbodorsal fascia or hamstrings, and traumatic sprains. Herniation of an intervertebral disc may produce localized neurologic signs or sciatic radiation of pain, but may also be associated with painless tight hamstrings alone.

Tumor. A neoplasm of the lower spinal cord may present with pain and localizing neurologic signs, as well as with a limp, paraparesis, or bladder dysfunction. In the adolescent, the most likely type of tumor to cause these symptoms is a lymphoma in the epidural space, although other tumors, such as a neurofibroma or glioma, may also occur. Further neurologic evaluation and magnetic resonance imaging (MRI) are indicated to define the location and extent of the lesion prior to surgical intervention or irradiation; the latter is often indicated for lymphomas.

Abscess. An epidural abscess shares certain clinical features of a spinal cord tumor, such as loss of bladder control and paraparesis, but the pain that accompanies it is much greater. The spine is typically held in rigid extension, and systemic signs of infection may be present. The causes include tuberculosis (resulting from extension from a site of vertebral osteomyelitis) or staphylococcus. The possibility of an epidural abscess should prompt immediate evaluation by MRI and neurosurgical consultation in order to prevent paraplegia. A pathologic skeletal condition, such as apophyseal fractures and spondylolysis, may also be responsible for low back pain in the adolescent. The latter is occurring with increasing frequency as more adolescents become athletically active. Particularly in sports such as gymnastics, recurrent flexion and extension of the spine are thought to cause stress fractures of the pars interarticularis, which are the underlying lesions in spondylolysis. A characteristic finding is pain on hyperextension; the diagnosis may be confirmed by technetium scanning.

Foot

Pain on the medial aspect associated with prominence of the head of the first metatarsal and lateral deviation of the great toe is found in hallux valgus (bunions), and is most common in adolescent girls.

Joints

Ankle

Examination of the adolescent with ankle pain requires systematic palpation in search of point tenderness. When this is found, it suggests ligamentous injury or fracture. Swelling is indicative of arthritis (infectious, collagen-vascular, Reiter syndrome) or osteochondritis dissecans.

Knee

Examination of the adolescent with pain in the knee and/or limp. The differential diagnosis includes recurrent dislocation of patella, osteochondritis dissecans, as well as the possibility of a pathologic condition of the hip or retroperitoneum. Sprains of the cruciate and/or collateral ligaments are first found during adolescence. A twisting force may cause avulsion of the anterior tibial spine, leading to rupture of anterior cruciate ligament. The presence of an effusion with a history of trauma suggests the possibility of a torn meniscus or ligament, osteochondral fracture, or posttraumatic synovitis. Effusion without trauma should prompt consideration of gonococcemia, Reiter syndrome, juvenile rheumatoid arthritis, or patellar malalignment.

Swelling below the patella, specifically at the tibial tubercle, is a common finding in Osgood-Schlatter disease.

Internal derangements are common with osteochondritis dissecans, causing osteochondral fractures. Locking of the knee may be secondary to tearing and meniscal displacement resulting from a torsion weight-bearing injury.

Trauma causing tenderness on both sides of the metaphysis of the femur suggests epiphyseal injury. Stress x-rays may reveal separation. The finding of a flexed knee in a patient with severe knee pain (usually a girl) suggests a recurrent dislocation of patella.

Hip

A history of a limp associated with pain in the hip or referred to the thigh or knee suggests the possibility of trauma, infection, malignancy, or systemic illness. Further history of systemic symptoms and of sexual activity must be obtained. Examination of the hip may reveal localized tenderness and hip flexion contraction with limitation of internal rotation. The differential diagnosis in the adolescent with these findings includes arthritis (secondary to collagen-vascular disease or gonococcemia) and slipped capital femoral epiphysis (SCFE).

It is important to perform a rectal examination in any adolescent with a limp or pain in the knee or hip, particularly if there are no findings at either of these sites. These conditions suggest referred or radiating pain from a retroperitoneal mass that is compressing the sacroiliac nerves.

Further evaluation includes x-rays in both the anteroposterior and lateral planes. In SCFE, the head of the femur is displaced posteriorly with separation through the proximal femoral epiphysis. There is, typically, limitation of abduction and internal rotation. Fracture or fluid in the joint space may be found, the latter suggesting either gonococcemia or collagen vascular disease.

X-ray Findings. Common radiographic findings in these bone lesions in the adolescent are as follows:

Osteochondroma:	Metaphyseal location in long bones Pedunculated or sessile Cartilage cap may be calcified
Osteoid osteoma:	Radiolucent lesion Approximately 1 cm in diameter surrounded by osteosclerosis
Osteoblastoma:	Nidus larger than 1 cm
Chondroblastoma:	Radiolucent lesion in ossification center with little or no reactive bone formation

Chondromyxofibroma:	Radiolucent, well-encapsulated lesion in long bone
Osteosarcoma and chondrosarcoma:	Radiolucent, destructive, invasive tumor with minimal host reaction may have ossification and/or calcification Metaphyseal location in long bones
Ewing's sarcoma:	Radiolucent, destructive lesion with active bone formation surrounding it in "onion-skin" arrangement. Found in diaphyseal region.

Long Bones

A history of **bone pain** in the adolescent suggests the following diagnoses:

Benign

- Osteoid osteoma and osteoblastoma—both present with increased pain at night that is relieved by acetylsalicylic acid (aspirin)
- Chondroma—may be associated with a pathologic fracture
- Chondroblastoma—the pain is usually close to a joint and may be associated with a pathologic fracture

Malignant

- Osteosarcoma and chondrosarcoma—pain is accompanied by a mass and, often, a pathologic fracture
- Ewing sarcoma—usually associated with tenderness, fever, leukocytosis, and a pathologic fracture

The finding of a painless **bone mass** suggests either a benign osteochondroma or chondromyxofibroma. The latter may be associated with a pathologic fracture.

NEUROLOGIC EXAMINATION

Muscle Strength

Puberty in males is associated not only with increase in muscle number and size, but also with increased strength. The peak of grip strength occurs shortly after the peak of the height velocity curve.

Muscle weakness may signify lesions of upper or lower motor neurons. Weakness of upper limb extensors and lower limb flexors is found with upper motor neuron lesions. Lower motor neuron lesions usually cause atrophy as well as weakness. If accompanied by fasciculations, anterior horn cell disease is likely. Distal weakness suggests peripheral nerve damage, and may be sign of chronic abuse of toluene or injection of a drug of abuse into a nerve.

Progressive symmetric proximal and distal weakness beginning in the legs and ascending to the thorax over the course of 3 days to 3 weeks, and associated with pain and paresthesias of the lower extremity, is the characteristic of Guillain-Barré syndrome (postinfectious polyneuritis).

Fine Motor Coordination. Tests such as those of rapid alternating supination and pronation of the hands should be performed easily by an adolescent. Failure to do so, such as slowing or irregularity, suggests cerebellar disease or abuse of alcohol or barbiturates.

Nystagmus. Disease of the cerebellum or brainstem, drugs, or a labyrinthine disturbance may account for the finding. The same disturbances that cause nystagmus may also cause **ataxia.**

Tremor. A tremor that is manifested when the patient reaches for an object or performs a finger-to-nose test, an **intention tremor,** suggests cerebellar dysfunction, which may result from the same causes as ataxia or nystagmus. A **fine tremor** upon trying to stretch fingers may be a sign of thyrotoxicosis, stimulant abuse, or withdrawal from narcotics or sedatives. A coarser **proximal tremor** (wing-beating tremor) is seen in Wilson disease.

Deep Tendon Reflexes

Hyperactive reflexes are found in upper motor neuron disease, hyperthyroidism, and in abuse of anticholinergics, stimulants, and hallucinogens (especially PCP).

Decreased or absent reflexes are seen in peripheral nerve or muscle disease or any condition that affects the reflex arc. Hypothyroidism, anorexia nervosa, and abuse of sedatives or narcotics are a few examples of this.

Extrapyramidal movements such as chorea, athetosis, and/or dystonia are signs of basal ganglia disease which, in the adolescent, is likely to be of toxic origin (for example, ingestion of the street drug contaminant MPTP or of antipsychotic drugs such as haloperidol). Rare heritable causes that may present during adolescence include Wilson disease, the late onset form of Hallervorden-Spatz disease, and Huntington disease. The fact that these abnormal movements disappear during sleep should not negate the possibility of organic disease.

Irregular jerking and writhing movement of the tongue, face, neck and/or upper extremity may be the only manifestation of acute rheumatic fever (Sydenham chorea) in the adolescent or may be precipitated by pregnancy. Huntington chorea is uncommon during adolescence, but 10% of cases have their onset at this time. The movement abnormalities typically occur before signs of dementia in this autosomal dominant condition.

Sensory Examination

Sensory deficits typically suggest peripheral nerve dysfunction. In hysterical sensory loss, the affected area stops at the midline, as opposed to that resulting from an organic lesion, which stops short of the midline by approximately 2.5 cm owing to overlap in innervation. Cutaneous hypersensitivity may be found over the distribution of a nerve irritated by infection with the herpes virus (zoster or type II) or by inflammation (over distribution of nerve involved in peritonitis) or trigeminal nerve distribution in posterior ethmoid sinusitis.

Cognitive Evaluation. See pp. 8–9.

Evaluation of Menstrual Dysfunction in the Adolescent

MENSTRUAL CRAMPS

Two-thirds of adolescent females experience menstrual cramps at some time, and nearly 15% suffer incapacitating dysmenorrhea. Thus, it is the leading cause of short-term school absenteeism among females. Despite the frequency and severity of menstrual cramps, most adolescent females believe that nothing can be done to alleviate their suffering and rarely seek help from a physician. With advances in understanding of its pathogenesis, however, it is now the exception that a patient with dysmenorrhea cannot be helped.

Dysmenorrhea is classified as primary or secondary. **Primary dysmenorrhea** occurs in the absence of any underlying organic disease. In this, the most common type of dysmenorrhea, the pain results from the stimulation of the myometrium by prostaglandins (F2 alpha and E2) produced in excessive amounts by the endometrium, which is sensitized by endogenously produced progesterone (from the corpus luteum following ovulation). By lowering prostaglandin levels (using cyclo-oxygenase inhibitors) or preventing ovulation (using conventional combination oral contraceptives), primary dysmenorrhea can be prevented or treated.

Secondary dysmenorrhea results from a structural or infectious process, such as endometriosis or endometritis, respectively (Table 24).

These two types of dysmenorrhea may be differentiated on the basis of history, physical examination, response to therapy, and, if necessary, laparoscopy (Fig. 11).

History

If pain occurs with the first menstrual period and if the flow is scant, consideration should be given to the possibility of partial cervical stenosis. In

TABLE 24. Causes of Secondary Dysmenorrhea

	Endometriosis	Endometritis
Pain		
Location	Pelvic	Pelvic
Pattern	Recurrent, with menses	Acute episode begins with menses, continues thereafter Pain may extend to involve entire abdomen, particularly right upper quadrant (perihepatitis)
Associated Findings	None	Fever Elevated WBC Elevated ESR Purulent discharge at onset
Pelvic Examination	Mild tenderness on palpation of involved area May have thickening, beading of rectovaginal septum and/or suspensory ligaments May find ovarian cyst ("chocolate") No vaginal discharge	Exquisite tenderness on palpation of uterus and on motion of cervix if fallopian tubes have become involved Purulent cervical discharge

most cases of primary dysmenorrhea, however, the history is that of onset of pain with subsequent, rather than the first, menstrual period. A history of fever or vaginal discharge suggests the possibility of endometritis, which is most likely due to a gonococcal infection in the adolescent who is not postpartum. Gonococcal infection typically ascends the genital tract from its cervical site of entry (initially as endometritis, followed by salpingitis, then possibly peritonitis and perihepatitis), with a menstrual period often confused with menstrual cramps. Chlamydia may behave in a similar manner but is less likely to produce symptomatic endometritis.

Physical Examination

Tenderness on cervical motion is diagnostic of salpingitis. Thickening of the rectovaginal septum or beading/thickening of the suspensory ligaments of the uterus suggests the diagnosis of endometriosis, although the examination may be negative and require laparoscopy to document its presence.

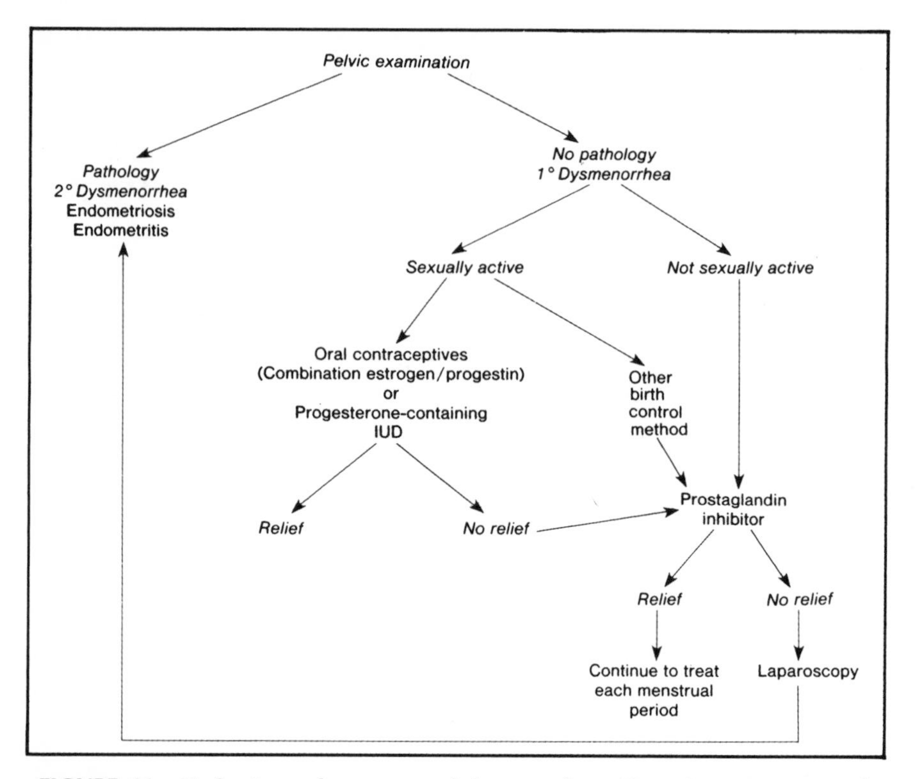

FIGURE 11. Evaluation and treatment of dysmenorrhea. (From Litt IF: Menstrual problems during adolescence. Pediatr Rev 4:203, 1983, with permission.)

Therapeutic Trial

Symptomatic response to prostaglandin inhibitors (such as sodium naproxen, 550 mg with onset of menses, and 275 mg every 6–8 hours thereafter for the first day of the menstrual period) is diagnostic of primary dysmenorrhea and requires no further evaluation. In the sexually active adolescent, it may be preferable to administer oral contraceptives (combination type, such as ethinyl estradiol/norethindrone) instead, as these will prevent endogenous production of progesterone and therefore preclude sensitization of the myometrium to the effects of the prostaglandins, decrease the amount of endometrial proliferation, and protect against unwanted pregnancy. Some mild cases of endometriosis may also respond to oral contraceptive therapy. Rarely, both an oral contraceptive and a prostaglandin inhibitor may be needed for a patient with primary dysmenorrhea.

Laparoscopy. If there is no response to prostaglandin inhibitors and/or oral contraceptives, the possibility of secondary dysmenorrhea should be entertained. Examination of the pelvic organs through a laparoscope is the least invasive (at the time of this writing) and most effective way of diagnosing endometriosis and other structural abnormalities of the uterus.

EXCESSIVE VAGINAL BLEEDING

Menometrorrhagia is one of the few emergency conditions that occur in adolescents and requires a prompt, sensitive, and effective response on the part of the primary care physician. A variety of systemic and local conditions may result in excessive vaginal bleeding (Table 25).

History

Because a congenital or acquired coagulopathy may produce menometrorrhegia, it is important to inquire about other bleeding manifestations (bruising, excessive bleeding with surgery or cuts, and so forth), although the most common of the congenital variety, von Willebrand disease, often presents for the first time at menarche. If massive bleeding occurs with the first menstrual period, serious consideration should be given to this

TABLE 25. Differential Diagnosis of Menometrorrhagia

Painless	Painful
Systemic	Trauma
Coagulopathy	Threatened abortion
Congenital	Salpingitis
von Willebrand disease	Intrauterine device
Acquired	
Aspirin sensitivity	
Aplastic anemia	
Anticoagulant treatment	
Neoplasm—bone marrow infiltration	
Idiopathic thrombocytopenia	
Endocrine	
Hypothyroidism	
Oral contraceptives—used improperly	
Local	
Gynecologic	
Dysfunctional uterine bleeding	
Neoplasm	

From Litt IF: Menstrual problems during adolescence. Pediatr Rev 4:203, 1983, with permission.

diagnosis, which can be confirmed by appropriate laboratory tests (for platelet adhesiveness and factor VIII level). These should be performed on blood drawn before any estrogen is given to stop the bleeding, as estrogen can increase the factor VIII level and thus possibly lead to the erroneous conclusion that it is normal (see below). The most common cause of an acquired coagulopathy is sensitivity to the acetyl moiety of acetylsalicylic acid (aspirin) taken in normal doses within 2 weeks before the bleeding episode. Thrombocytopenia that results from bone marrow replacement by a tumor, aplasia, or hypoplasia is a less common cause of menometrorrhagia. Other symptoms of hypothyroidism should be sought, but it is not uncommon for excessive menstrual bleeding to be the first indication of this disorder. Erratic use of oral contraceptives by adolescents who think that contraceptives are to be taken "PRN" accounts for some cases of excessive (in this case, withdrawal) bleeding. The most common explanation for menometrorrhagia in the young adolescent is so-called dysfunctional uterine bleeding, the result of endometrial buildup and subsequent uncontrollable shedding in anovulatory patients who lack progesterone to counteract the effects of estrogen. Accordingly, a history of the timing of last menstrual period should be taken. Typically, there has been a long interval between the last period and the problematic period.

Painful, heavy vaginal bleeding may result from a threatened abortion, the presence of an intrauterine device, or salpingitis. A sensitive interview will establish whether the patient is sexually active and if any of these diagnoses may be the cause of the bleeding. Trauma may also cause heavy vaginal bleeding and may result from a sports-related injury (such as water skiing) or intercourse (first or forceful), the latter possibility again requiring sensitive and confidential inquiry.

Physical Examination

In the patient with a history of heavy vaginal bleeding, the first task is to establish the extent of blood loss in order to determine the course of management. Vital signs are taken immediately to detect the presence of hypovolemic shock. If pulse and blood pressure (including orthostatic determinations) are normal, the subsequent examination focuses on establishing the cause of the bleeding. To rule out the possibility that it is secondary to a coagulopathy, the trunk should be examined for ecchymoses and/or petechiae. Examination should also focus on the possibility that a coagulopathy may be the result of marrow replacement by tumor, and hence evidence of enlarged lymph nodes, liver, and/or spleen is sought. The thyroid gland should be palpated, and the texture of the hair and skin noted, as these are more subtle signs of hypothyroidism, another possible cause of menometrorrhagia. The presence of fever may suggest the possibility of endometritis/salpingitis, which may be associated with acute onset of increased menstrual bleeding. Increased pigmentation of the areola or linea alba suggests that the patient may be pregnant and experiencing a threatened abortion. The pelvic examination will help to determine the etiology of the bleeding by revealing the presence of lacerations, a foul odor, or enlarged uterus, the first being indicative of trauma; the second, of endometritis/salpingitis; and the last, of pregnancy. The finding of a soft, cyanotic cervix is also compatible with the diagnosis of pregnancy, but is insufficiently specific and reliable to warrant the risk of performing this procedure in someone suspected of having a threatened abortion. The finding of an adenexal mass suggests the possibility of an ovarian tumor, whereas adenexal tenderness on cervical motion indicates salpingitis.

Laboratory Tests

1. Pregnancy test (beta subunit HCG)
2. Complete blood count
3. Type and cross-match
4. Thyroid function tests (T4, T3, TSH)
5. Bleeding time
6. Clotting time
7. Platelet count
8. Factor VIII level
9. Test of platelet adhesiveness

Draw blood for #4 and #8 before administering estrogen. If the patient is hemorrhaging and/or appears to be in shock, blood should be drawn through the intravenous line established to replace and maintain intravascular volume.

Management

Although management is not the focus of this book, in the case of menometrorrhagia, the treatment intervention may be diagnostic as well as therapeutic, and is therefore included. Administration of a combination of estrogen and progesterone, in the doses provided in Enovid, will stop bleeding due to anything other than trauma, pregnancy, and salpingitis within 2 hours of administration of 25 mg. The subsequent treatment regimen is outlined in Figure 12.

AMENORRHEA

Primary amenorrhea refers to the absence of menses in an individual who has never menstruated (i.e., not achieved menarche by the age-appropriate time). The point at which a patient should be considered to have primary amenorrhea is not absolute, as the normal age range for achieving menarche is quite broad. Menarche may occur as early as 10 years or as late

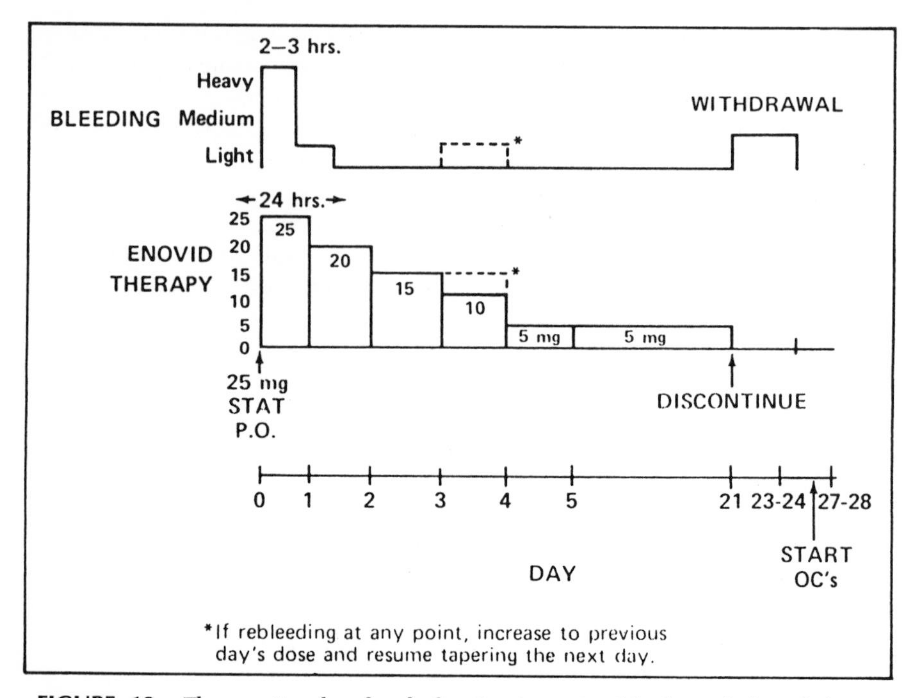

FIGURE 12. Therapeutic plan for dysfunctional uterine bleeding. (Adapted from Altchek A: Dysfunctional menstrual disorders in adolescence. Clin Obstet Gynecol 14:975, 1971, with permission.)

as 16 years and still be within the "normal" range. Better than population norms, however, is the patient's own family history, as there is excellent concordance between mothers' and their daughters' (and even better between siblings') ages at menarche. If a young women is more than 1 year older than was her mother or sister when either experienced menarche, she should be considered to have primary amenorrhea, even if she falls within the "normal" age range for the larger population. Similarly, the relationship between progression of pubertal development and menarche is so consistent that it is appropriate to consider a young woman who is 13 years old and has not reached SMR 2 as having primary amenorrhea. A young woman who has begun pubertal development but in whom there has been failure of progression for a period of more than 2 years should also be considered in the same context.

Secondary amenorrhea refers to absence of monthly menses of more than 3 months' duration in a previously menstruating female.

Differential Diagnosis

The etiologies of primary and secondary amenorrhea in the adolescent may be considered together (Table 26), except that in the former congenital and chromosomal anomalies must be included with other conditions that may be responsible for both forms of amenorrhea.

Congenital Anomalies. Between 20 and 40% of cases of primary amenorrhea are caused by congenital abnormalities, such as failure of normal development of the mullerian duct system (for example, imperforate hymen, vaginal agenesis, cervical stenosis, or uterine agenesis) or chromosomal abnormalities (such as gonadal dysgenesis, Turner syndrome, or testicular feminization). Abnormalities of the mullerian duct system are generally isolated findings, whereas the chromosomal abnormalities that cause amenorrhea characteristically result in other anomalies as well.

Turner Syndrome (XO Karyotype or Mosaicism). This syndrome is characterized by the presence of dysgenetic, undifferentiated gonads, short stature, and, often, webbed neck and widely spaced nipples. It is the most common of the chromosomal anomalies that cause amenorrhea and is among the leading causes of this condition in an older adolescent female at SMR 1 or 2. In the absence of the normal suppressive action of ovarian estradiol and progesterone on the pituitary gland, gonadotropin levels are markedly elevated. The earlier the diagnosis is made, the better, as administration of exogenous estrogens and progestins will permit breast development and

TABLE 26. Differential Diagnosis of Amenorrhea

- Congenital anomalies
  - Gonads (Turner syndrome, testicular feminization syndrome)
  - Mullerian duct system (vaginal agenesis, imperforate hymen, cervical stenosis, uterine agenesis)
- Chronic illness (see Table 27)
- Psychogenic
  - Anorexia nervosa
  - Stress
  - Pseudocyesis
- Drugs (see Table 28)
- Endocrine
  - Hypothalamic dysfunction (tumor, weight loss, athletics)
  - Panhypopituitarism (craniopharyngioma, prolactinoma)
  - Hypogonadotropic hypogonadism (Kallmann syndrome)
  - Thyroid dysfunction (hypo- or hypersecretion)
  - Adrenal dysfunction (hypo- or hypersecretion)
- Gynecologic
  - Ovarian
    - Tumor
    - Cyst
    - Polycystic ovary
  - Uterine
    - Pregnancy
    - Endometrial hypoplasia

From Litt IF: Menstrual problems during adolescence. Pediatr Rev 4:203, 1983, with permission.

monthly withdrawal bleeding from a uterus that is typically normal in this syndrome, and will help to prevent osteoporosis.

Chronic Illness. Retardation of pubertal development and, hence, delay in menarche may result from any chronic illness that interferes with hypothalamic-pituitary-ovarian function, directly or indirectly, particularly in instances in which the illness compromises tissue oxygenation or nutrition. If the chronic illness is acquired after completion of pubertal development and menarche, secondary amenorrhea may result instead. Examples of these categories are found in Table 27.

Drugs. Both illicit and prescribed medications may cause amenorrhea by a variety of mechanisms in the adolescent: by suppressing gonadotropin-releasing hormone GnRH (either directly or indirectly), by affecting dopamine or endorphin levels, by inhibiting prolactin-inhibiting factor (PIF), or by having direct toxic effect on the ovaries. Some of these drugs may also cause galactorrhea or a false-positive pregnancy test. A list of drugs that may cause amenorrhea is included in Table 28.

Psychogenic Conditions. Emotional stress may cause amenorrhea. The younger the person, the more likely it is that amenorrhea will occur under stressful conditions. Leaving home for the first time, the so-called boarding school syndrome, is the most common manifestation of this phenomenon. The stress of competition has been proposed as a mechanism for the amenorrhea associated with competitive athletics, but this is not universally accepted. The impact of emotional stress on menstrual function is likely mediated through the suppressive effect of increased levels of neurotransmitters on GnRH. The high frequency with which evidence of stress is found in the lives of most adolescents, with or without amenorrhea,

TABLE 27. Chronic Illnesses That May Cause Amenorrhea

Direct Endocrine Effect
Hypothalamic tumor
Pituitary insufficiency (or tumor)
Thyroid disease (hypersecretion or, rarely, hyposecretion)
Adrenal (insufficiency or hypersecretion)
Sickle cell anemia
Thalassemia major
Diabetes mellitus (in poor control)
Compromised Tissue Oxygenation
Cyanotic congenital heart disease
Cystic fibrosis
Compromised Nutrition
Inflammatory bowel disease
Cystic fibrosis
Anorexia nervosa

From Litt IF: Menstrual problems during adolescence. Pediatr Rev 4:203, 1983, with permission.

makes it mandatory to explore all possible causes when amenorrhea is present. Organic etiologies should be considered before assuming that the presence of stress is causally related to the amenorrhea.

Anorexia nervosa is a well-recognized psychogenic condition in which amenorrhea is a universal finding. Although it commonly presents with secondary amenorrhea, 25% of our patients with anorexia nervosa have manifested primary amenorrhea. Malnutrition plays an important role in its pathogenesis, but one-third to one-half of patients with anorexia nervosa develop amenorrhea months before significant weight loss occurs and fail to resume menses when they regain their pre-morbid weight. The longest delays in menstrual resumption (up to 4 years after weight rehabilitation) are associated with continued psychiatric disturbance and/or strenuous athletics.

Pseudocyesis, a condition in which amenorrhea is associated with symptoms of pregnancy and a protuberant abdomen, is rare in adolescents. When these symptoms are found in a teenager with a negative pregnancy test, this diagnosis should be considered and psychiatric consultation sought.

Endocrinologic Abnormalities. Hypopituitarism in the adolescent is most often secondary to a tumor, the most common of which is a craniopharyngioma. Its discovery is typically prompted by delay in pubertal development and/or primary amenorrhea. The skull x-ray finding of suprasellar calcifications confirms the diagnosis, but its absence does not rule it out. The associated finding of galactorrhea suggests the possibility of a prolactinoma, although this tumor may present with secondary amenorrhea alone. A skull x-ray may demonstrate an enlarged or asymmetric pituitary fossa, but it may also be normal. A CT scan or MRI should be performed if a prolactinoma is suspected. Because it has been demonstrated that galactorrhea and amenorrhea may antedate roentgenographic evidence of a tumor by more than 10 years, it may be necessary to be even more aggressive in its pursuit (see Laboratory Evaluation on p. 111).

Disturbances of production of specific gonadotropins may result from a variety of hypothalamic as well as pituitary abnormalities. For example, loss of the normal pubertal pulsatile or sleep-augmented secretory pattern of production of GnRH by the hypothalamus may result from weight loss of as little as 10% of body weight or from strenuous exercise, and may cause abnormally low levels of LH with amenorrhea. Suppression of GnRH by medications or stress may produce the same end result. Hypogonadotropic hypogonadism (Kallmann syndrome) is characterized by blunted or absent ability to perceive certain odors (such as coffee or perfume), lack of pubertal development with primary amenorrhea, low serum levels of LH, and normal ovarian response to exogenously administered gonadotropins.

Abnormalities of other pituitary target organs, such as the thyroid and adrenal glands, may also result in amenorrhea. Among these, hyperthyroidism is the most common. It is postulated that the suppressive effect of high levels of thyroxine on pituitary TSH is similarly suppressive of gonadotropin production. Interestingly, however, hypothyroidism that occurs prior to puberty may result in primary amenorrhea. Congenital adrenal hyperplasia, if mild, may first present during adolescence with amenorrhea and evidence of virilization, both of which are reversible with replacement therapy. Cushing syndrome may cause delayed puberty or secondary amenorrhea, its presentation depending on the timing of its occurrence.

Ovarian Disease. Ovarian disease may cause amenorrhea, as in the case of Turner syndrome, or as a result of the effects of certain chemotherapeutic agents. In addition, amenorrhea may result from estrogen-producing tumors such as a dermoid cyst or those that produce androgen, such as an arrhenoblastoma or lipid cell tumor. The latter may cause masculinizing effects in addition to amenorrhea. Another pathologic condition of the ovary (which may actually reflect pituitary dysfunction rather than primary ovarian pathology) that commonly produces adolescent amenorrhea is the polycystic ovarian syndrome (Stein-Leventhal). It is the most common cause of amenorrhea in patients who have completed pubertal development (SMR 5). In contrast to older women with this syndrome, adolescents, presumably because they have as yet had little exposure to the associated elevated testosterone levels, rarely are masculinized or obese. The diagnosis is occasionally suggested by palpation of enlarged ovaries, or ultrasonographic demonstration of cysts—inconsistent findings in this age group. The diagnosis is confirmed by the documentation of marked elevation in LH levels in the presence of normal FSH levels ($\geq$ 3:1). Use of combination oral contraceptive therapy is desirable to lower testosterone levels and, presumably, to prevent the masculinizing sequelae previously thought to be an invariable component of the syndrome.

Uterine Causes. As menses represents shedding of the endometrium, any condition that interferes with this process will cause amenorrhea. The most common of these is pregnancy, a diagnosis that is often not considered as readily in adolescents as in adult women. Although pregnancy most commonly causes secondary amenorrhea, many adolescents have become pregnant before ever experiencing menarche (hence, primary amenorrhea)! Much rarer uterine causes of amenorrhea are endometrial hypoplasia or synechiae (Asherman syndrome), which may result from repeated curettage of the uterus or from irradiation. Relative hypoplasia may occur following discontinuation of oral contraceptives, "post-pill" amenorrhea, which may continue for up to 18 months in adolescents.

History

Family History. In order to establish if a patient suspected of having primary amenorrhea qualifies for this diagnostic designation, it is useful to learn the age of menarche of the patient's mother and sisters. If the patient is more than one year older than they were at their menarche, she should be considered to have primary amenorrhea, regardless of her stage of pubertal development or of being within the population norms for menarcheal age.

Sexual History. The possibility of pregnancy must always be considered in patients with either primary or secondary amenorrhea. Obtaining a sensitive and confidential sexual history is mandatory in order to establish the diagnosis expeditiously and without unnecessary testing for other conditions (see p. 21–27).

Drug History. As indicated above, a number of prescribed and illicit drugs may cause amenorrhea (Table 28). A drug history must be taken.

History of Weight Loss and Exercise. Weight loss of as little as 10%, or excessive strenuous exercise, or both are commonly associated with amenorrhea. The possibility of anorexia nervosa should also be considered in such cases. When weight loss and amenorrhea occur in the absence of voluntary restriction of food, organic illness (such as hyperthyroidism, inflammatory bowel disease, or diabetes mellitus) or depression should be suspected.

History of Timing and Patterns of Landmarks of Physical Growth and Development. If secondary sex characteristics have not appeared by the

TABLE 28. Drugs That May Cause Amenorrhea

- Illicit Drugs
  - Heroin
  - Methadone
  - Marijuana
- Prescribed Drugs
  - Hormones
    - Oral contraceptives (estrogen and progesterone combinations or progestins alone)
    - Progestins
    - Testosterone
    - Danazol
  - Antihypertensives
    - Methyldopa
  - Antidepressants
    - Phenothiazines
  - Vitamins
    - Vitamin A (in toxic doses)
  - Chemotherapeutic agents
    - Cyclophosphamide
    - Chlorambucil
    - Vincaleukoblastine
    - Methylhydrazine
  - Radioisotopes
    - ^{32}P
    - ^{131}I
    - ^{198}Au

From Litt IF: Menstrual problems during adolescence. Pediatr Rev 4:203, 1983, with permission.

age of 13 years, a chromosomal abnormality, chronic illness, or craniopharyngioma should be suspected. Lack of progression of development of secondary sex characteristics suggests an acquired condition.

History of Headache or Visual Disturbance. A positive history will suggest a central nervous system tumor as the cause of the amenorrhea.

History of Abdominal Pain. If midline lower abdominal pain occurs in association with primary amenorrhea in a young woman with age-appropriate development of secondary sex characteristics, it is likely that an anomaly of the mullerian duct structures (such as imperforate hymen with resultant hematocolpos or cervical stenosis with resultant hematometrium) is responsible. Unilateral abdominal pain would be more suggestive of an ovarian tumor.

History of Abnormal Hair Development or Acne. An increase in the appearance or pigmentation of body hair, development of facial hair, or severe acne suggest an androgen-producing ovarian tumor, adrenal hypersecretion, or polycystic ovaries. As previously noted, however, the last may occur without any signs of masculinization.

History of Galactorrhea. A prolactin-secreting adenoma or pregnancy may cause of galactorrhea. (See pp. 77–79 for further discussion of galactorrhea.)

Psychosocial Assessment. Emotional stress may cause amenorrhea, and anorexia nervosa invariably does. It is important that these possibilities be explored through history taking. The discovery of stress is not, in and of itself, diagnostic of the cause of amenorrhea, as stress may also be present in a patient with an organic cause of her amenorrhea.

Physical Examination

General Appearance. Emaciation suggests either a severe chronic illness, such as inflammatory bowel disease or cystic fibrosis, or anorexia nervosa. A flat affect or lack of eye contact may indicate use of an illicit or prescribed psychoactive drug, or depression, or both. Short stature suggests the possibility of chromosomal anomaly or delay in the pubertal growth spurt. Cyanotic congenital heart disease or cystic fibrosis may cause amenorrhea, so the finding of cyanosis may be informative.

Vital Signs. *Pulse.* Bradycardia is found in patients with anorexia nervosa, conditioned athletes (not typically less than 45/min), or increased intracranial pressure. The pulse is elevated in hyperthyroidism.

Blood Pressure. Low blood pressure (particularly with postural changes) is found in anorexia nervosa. Elevated blood pressure suggests increased intracranial pressure or adrenal hypersecretion. Wide pulse-pressure occurs in hyperthyroidism.

Temperature. Body temperature is low in anorexia nervosa and elevated in hyperthyroidism and inflammatory bowel disease.

HEENT. Pupillary changes and nystagmus suggest drug use. Blurred discs suggest increased intracranial pressure, usually secondary to a central nervous system tumor. Subconjunctival hemorrhage with or without pharyngeal lacerations may be found in anorexia nervosa with bulimic features. Parotid swelling without fever is another clue to recurrent vomiting.

Neck. Enlarged thyroid gland is found in hyperthyroidism, although most goiters in adolescent females are euthyroid and associated with thyroiditis, not usually a cause of amenorrhea. A webbed neck is found in Turner syndrome.

Chest. Wide-spaced nipples may be found in Turner syndrome. Galactorrhea is a sign of a prolactin-secreting tumor or of pregnancy, the latter also being associated with increased pigmentation of the areola and enlargement of the tubercles of Montgomery. Stage of development of breasts should also be ascertained in order to determine if puberty is delayed or age-appropriate.

Cardiac. Cyanotic congenital heart disease may cause primary amenorrhea.

Abdomen. The finding of a mass in the lower abdomen may indicate hematocolpos, hematometrium, or pregnant uterus if in the midline, and an ovarian neoplasm if unilateral.

Genitalia. Stage of development of pubic hair will assist in determining the cause of amenorrhea. If puberty is at the age-appropriate stage, then a diagnosis of chromosomal abnormality can usually be excluded. Clitoral hypertrophy suggests an androgen-secreting ovarian tumor or adrenal hyperplasia. A bulging, bluish hymen is diagnostic of imperforate hymen. The presence of the cervix should be established by digital-bimanual or rectal-bimanual examination. A soft, cyanotic cervix and a midline mass suggest pregnancy.

Skin. Lanugo hair on the trunk and back and dry skin are common findings in anorexia nervosa. Facial hair and increased pigmentation of body hair and acne are seen in adrenal hyperplasia, androgen-secreting ovarian tumor, and polycystic ovary syndrome. Increased pigmentation of the linea alba and areolae are signs of pregnancy.

Neurologic Examination. This is performed to rule out the possibility that amenorrhea is the result of a central nervous system tumor (the most common of which are craniopharyngioma and prolactinoma) or of illicit drug abuse.

Laboratory Tests

An algorithm for approaching the diagnostic evaluation of the patient with amenorrhea is found in Figure 13.

Pregnancy Test. Serum beta-HCG should be measured in all cases of secondary amenorrhea, regardless of history. It should also be measured in selected patients with primary amenorrhea, particularly in those with advanced pubertal development.

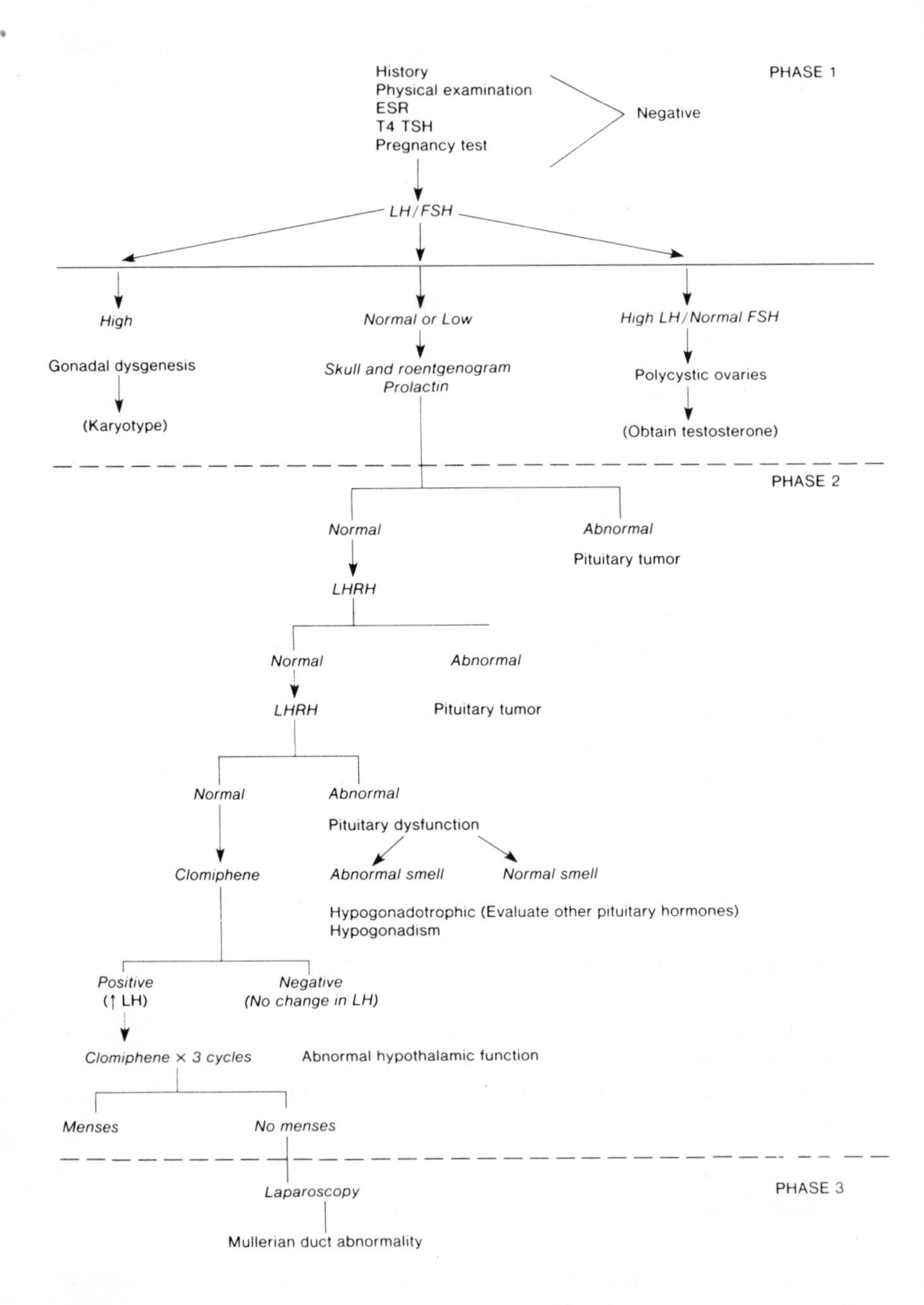

FIGURE 13. Evaluation of adolescent amenorrhea. (From Litt IF: Menstrual problems during adolescence. Pediatr Rev 4:203, 1983, with permission.)

Hematocrit. Iron deficiency anemia may be etiologically related to amenorrhea. A low hematocrit may also represent the presence of a chronic disease that is responsible for the amenorrhea.

Erythrocyte Sedimentation Rate (ESR). An elevated ESR suggests that a chronic illness, such as inflammatory bowel disease, may be responsible for the amenorrhea. An extremely low ESR (for example, less than 4 mm/hr) may suggest anorexia nervosa.

Serum FSH and LH. Normal values are listed in Appendix 8, pp. 197–201. High levels are diagnostic of gonadal dysgenesis. Low or normal levels may be found with a pituitary tumor, hypogonadotropic hypogonadism, hypothalamic or pituitary dysfunction (such as is often found in patients with anorexia nervosa or endurance athletes), or mullerian duct abnormality. When a pituitary neoplasm has been ruled out by appropriate radiologic study (see below), an LHRH stimulation test, followed by administration of clomiphene, will permit differentiation between pituitary and hypothalamic dysfunction and structural abnormalities of the internal genitalia. A high level of LH and normal FSH is a pattern diagnostic of polycystic ovarian syndrome.

Serum Prolactin Level. A normal level is less than 20 ng/ml. An elevated level is a diagnostic of a prolactin-secreting tumor of the pituitary, although normal levels do not rule out this possibility.

Thyroid Function Tests. Because either hypothyroidism or hyperthyroidism may cause amenorrhea, T3, T4, and TSH levels should be obtained. These are all low in anorexia nervosa.

17-Ketosteroids. These levels may be elevated in the patient with adrenal hyperplasia or in one-third of those with polycystic ovary syndrome.

Radiologic Studies

If there is difficulty palpating the cervix, uterus, or ovaries, ultrasonography of the pelvis may be helpful.

Lateral skull x-ray may reveal calcifications in the suprasellar area caused by a craniopharyngioma. An enlarged sella is also suggestive of a pituitary tumor. A negative skull x-ray does not, however, rule out the possibility of an intracranial neoplasm, and other tests (see below) may be necessary.

CT scan or MRI may detect prolactinoma (adenoma) or other central nervous system tumor.

Other Test Procedures

Medroxyprogesterone acetate (Provera) is often administered in the evaluation of patients with amenorrhea. The occurrence of withdrawal bleeding following its use indicates that the patient has a uterus, a patent cervix, and is sufficiently estrogenized to have a proliferative endometrium. If this agent is used, it should be given after blood has been drawn for other endocrinologic determinations, and after a pregnancy test is found to be negative.

If the above evaluation fails to elucidate the etiology of the amenorrhea, laparoscopy to visualize the mullerian duct system, and possibly an ovarian biopsy, should be considered.

Evaluation of the Adolescent with Headaches

The differential diagnosis of headaches in the adolescent patient is found in Table 29.

History

Chronicity. The rapidity with which a diagnostic evaluation should be undertaken largely reflects the acuity of the headache. Recent onset of headaches that are excruciatingly painful or associated with fever and/or head trauma is an indication for immediate evaluation to rule out potentially life-threatening conditions. The evaluation of the chronic headache may be done over a more protracted period of time and may be assisted by the patient's keeping a pain diary. Entries should include the date, time of day, and duration of the headache, as well as activities, stresses, or other symptoms that occur at the time, and activities or medications that relieved the symptoms.

Family History. The history of a family member with headaches is useful information, both in terms of the familial nature of migraine and of the possibility of role modeling in a conversion reaction. Families with migraine are more likely to have members who suffer from motion sickness or from "ice cream" headaches.

Associated Symptoms. Migraine and vascular headaches are often preceded by a visual aura (scintillating scotoma or bright lights) and accompanied by nausea, vomiting, vertigo, and/or photophobia. Uncommonly, there may be transient neurologic aberrations, such as micropsia and metamorphopsia (distortions in size, shapes, and spatial relationships of objects), aphasia, hemiplegia, ophthalmoplegia, or paresthesias. The finding of localized and persistent neurologic symptoms and/or a seizure should prompt concern about the possibility of a vascular malformation or brain

TABLE 29. Differential Diagnosis of Headaches in the Adolescent

Vascular
Classic migraine
Ophthalmoplegic migraine
Basilar migraine
Cluster headache
Trauma
Postconcussion syndrome
Subdural hematoma
Neoplastic
Arteriovenous malformation
Central nervous system leukemia
Tumor
Infectious
Brain abscess
Sinusitis
Dental abscess
Collagen-vascular
JRA temporomandibular joint
Systemic lupus erythematosus
Barometric
Systemic hypertension
Pseudotumor cerebri
Psychogenic
Tension
Conversion reaction
Hypochondriasis

tumor. Patients with functional/tension headaches, on the other hand, may report lightheaded dizziness, but not true vertigo. Vomiting with a headache of increasing severity suggests the possibility of increased intracranial pressure, as may result from a neoplasm or pseudotumor cerebri. Diplopia may occur in association with central nervous system leukemia, pseudotumor cerebri, and other neoplasms. A history of high fever should prompt consideration of meningitis.

Location. Migraine headaches tend to be well-localized and are often unilateral. Tension headaches may be poorly localized or limited to the vertex. Frontal headaches suggest sinusitis. The pain associated with a brain tumor may not be well-localized. A headache in the temporal area may be a symptom of a dental abscess or of involvement of the temporomandibular joint in juvenile rheumatoid arthritis.

Character of the Pain. The pain of migraine is typically throbbing, and in tension headaches is generally dull. Patients with conversion reactions tend to describe their headaches in dramatic and vivid terms, although their affect remains rather bland.

Pattern. Migraine or vascular headaches tend to occur in paroxyms or attacks, separated by trouble-free intervals. Migraines are usually relieved by sleep, but other vascular headaches may awaken the patient from sleep. Tension headaches, on the other hand, are reported to be constant and occur daily for long periods of time. A headache that occurs only on weekdays and keeps the adolescent out of school may be symptomatic of school avoidance. Persistence with worsening over the course of several weeks suggests increased intracranial pressure or hypertension.

Response to Medication. Migraine will respond to appropriate medication, whereas a tension headache is often resistant to all medications.

History of Head Trauma. The postconcussion syndrome may be manifested by chronic headaches without any physical findings. There may or may not be associated symptoms of hyperacusis, dizziness, and emotional lability. Of greater seriousness is a subdural hematoma, which should be suspected if headache, stiff neck, focal neurologic signs, or personality change is noted after a period of apparent recovery from the head trauma.

Physical Examination

General Appearance. Patients with tension headaches generally appear physically well or depressed, their complaints notwithstanding. Those with migraine, meningitis, or brain tumor appear acutely ill.

Vital Signs. Elevated temperature should prompt consideration of the possibility of encephalitis or meningitis. Thermal instability may suggest a hypothalamic neoplasm. Elevated blood pressure may be the cause of the headache, in and of itself, or a sign of increased intracranial pressure, the latter typically being accompanied by bradycardia. A wide pulse-pressure in the adolescent with a headache may point to an arteriovenous malformation as the cause of both.

HEENT. Tenderness or lack of transillumination of the sinuses suggests sinusitis as the cause of headache. Tenderness upon tapping of the upper molars is compatible with a dental abscess, which may present with a headache. Examination of the visual fields and eye grounds is necessary to identify a field cut or papilledema, either of which mandates immediate CT scan or MRI to rule out the possibility of a CNS neoplasm. Unilateral conjunctival injection, lacrimation, and rhinorrhea may be found in patients with cluster headaches.

Neck. Stiffness and pain on neck flexion in a patient with fever may be indicative of meningitis or encephalitis and necessitate immediate evaluation. Spasticity of the sternocleidomastoid muscles in the adolescent with a generalized or occipital headache is compatible with a tension headache.

Neurologic Examination. In addition to examination of the eye grounds for signs of papilledema, it is important that any localizing neurologic signs be identified, as they suggest the presence of a neoplasm, ophthalmoplegic migraine, subdural hematoma, or vascular malformation. In the febrile patient with a headache and stiff neck, the neurologic examination may yield additional evidence of encephalitis or meningitis (such as positive Kernig and Brudinski signs). In hemiplegic migraine, there may be hemiparesis, paresthesias, or hemisensory loss that precedes the occurrence of a headache on the contralateral side by hours to days. Meningeal signs in the afebrile patient with an excruciating headache suggest rupture of an intracranial aneurysm, a true emergency. In basilar artery migraine, there may be sudden onset of ataxia, circumoral and distal extremity paresthesias, and cranial nerve deficits.

Skin. The presence of café-au-lait spots, areas of increased or decreased pigmentation, hemangiomata, vascular nevi, or other vascular signs suggest the possibility of a neurocutaneous syndrome and, with it, that of a central nervous system tumor or vascular malformation as the cause of the headaches.

Mental Status. See pp. 47–49.

Laboratory Evaluation

Electroencephalogram. Unless the headache is associated with a seizure, the EEG is not likely to be useful. Approximately 15% of adolescents have nonspecific EEG abnormalities of no clinical significance.

CT Scan or MRI. In the presence of localizing neurologic signs, signs of increased intracranial pressure, or excruciating pain, these tests may be useful in identifying a neoplasm, vascular anomaly, subdural hematoma, or pseudotumor cerebri.

Therapeutic Trial. If relief from a headache with symptoms and signs of classic migraine is achieved by use of a combination of ergotamine tartrate and caffeine, the diagnosis is confirmed. Failure to obtain relief from these pharmacologic agents does not, however, rule out the possibility that the headache is a migraine.

Evaluation of the Adolescent with Chest Pain

Chest pain is a common cause of disability, school absence, and doctor visits among adolescents. The differential diagnosis of this symptom is outlined in Table 30. Although the list is quite extensive, the most common causes of chest pain in the adolescent are musculoskeletal, psychogenic, (including hyperventilation), or breast-related. The location of the pain, as provided in the table, is not as useful in establishing the etiology as it is in the adult patient. Regardless of the actual cause of the pain, most teenagers with chest pain imagine the worst and are often worried that they have cancer or are having a heart attack. In a study by Pantell, it was documented that nearly one-third of adolescents with chest pain had experienced negative life events within the 6 months prior to onset of their pain. Of interest was a lack of relationship between the experience of negative life events and the specific diagnosis. This suggests that consideration be given to the possible need for supportive therapy, regardless of the actual diagnosis made.

CHEST PAIN

Cardiac Causes

Fear of a heart attack is common in adolescents who have chest pain, particularly those who have previously been given any cardiac diagnosis (including "functional" heart murmur) or who have relatives who have actually experienced a myocardial infarct. The rarity of infarction in this age group notwithstanding, a few conditions may predispose to this event, including chronic illnesses such as sickle cell anemia and muscular dystrophy, congenital abnormalities such as aberrant coronary artery or type 2 hyperlipidemia, acute conditions such as vasculitides (for example, systemic

TABLE 30. Chest Pain in the Adolescent

System	Location	Quality	Associated Findings
Cardiac			
Arrhythmias	Substernal, neck	Fluttering	Pallor, sweating, anxiety
Pericarditis	Sternum or over apex with radiation to neck and left arm	Acute onset, stabbing	Fever Pericardial friction rub, pulsus paradoxus
Mitral valve prolapse	Apical	Pressure is angina-like	Palpitations, mid-systolic click, late systolic murmur, skeletal abnormalities
Severe aortic stenosis	Retrosternal	Angina-like worsens with exertion	In aortic area—systolic ejection murmur and thrill
Hypertrophic subaortic stenosis			Delayed-onset crescendo decrescendo systolic murmur, middle left to upper right sternal border with a systolic thrill; a double or triple apical impulse (precordial ripple) may be seen or palpated
Pulmonary			
Pulmonary embolism	At site of infarction	Sudden onset, sharp or dull, worsened by inspiration	Tachypnea, tachycardia, hypotension, pleural rub
Pleurisy	At site of consolidation	Pleuritic pain with breathing	May have pleural rub and findings of pneumonia (cough, fever, dyspnea, rales, bronchial breath sounds)
Spontaneous pneumothorax	Unilateral	Sudden onset, sharp and well-localized, worsened by breathing	Hyperresonance, dyspnea, decreased breath sounds

TABLE 30. Chest Pain in the Adolescent *(Continued)*

System	Location	Quality	Associated Findings
Breast			Gynecomastia, use of oral contraceptives Time in cycle Fear of breast cancer
Musculoskeletal			
Muscle strain	Localized	Aching	
Costochondritis	Localized		Swelling of costochondral junction, worsened by movement
Gastrointestinal			
Esophagitis	Lower sternum	Gradual onset of burning, worsens when lying down	
Esophageal tear (rupture)	Substernal or pain in neck	Sudden, burning	Crepitus if pneumomediastinum
Psychogenic	May be localized to region thought to be the heart	Usually transient, may migrate and be sharp	Tenderness to palpation May be hyperventilation History of heart disease in family

lupus erythematosus), mucocutaneous lymph node syndrome (Kawasaki disease), infective endocarditis, and use of cocaine. Other cardiac causes of chest pain in adolescents are as follows.

Arrhythmias. The pain associated with an arrhythmia, most commonly premature ventricular contractions (PVCs), may be bounding or fluttering, or experienced as a skipped beat. This may be experienced substernally or in the neck, and is the result of the increased cardiac output in the normal beat that follows a compensatory pause. PVCs may occur in isolation or may be precipitated by fever, caffeine, or other stimulants, or by anxiety. Regardless of its precipitant, it may be accompanied by pallor, sweating, and anxiety.

Pericarditis. The pain of pericardial disease is acute in onset and experienced as sharp and stabbing. It is precordial and may radiate to the left shoulder, neck, and back, and is often worsened by lying down and relieved by sitting forward. This pain is believed to be referred from the diaphragm and pleura. The patient appears acutely ill. Fever and cough may be present, depending on the cause, which includes viral, bacterial (e.g., tuberculous), fungal, or parasitic infections, inflammatory processes (e.g., systemic lupus erythematosus or acute rheumatic fever), trauma, and postpericardiotomy syndrome. In adolescents, as much as a liter of fluid may accumulate in the pericardial sac, with signs related to the amount of fluid present. For example, a friction rub may be apparent with small amounts of fluid, whereas the presence of neck vein distention, pulsus paradoxus, and distant heart sounds suggest that large amounts of fluid have accumulated.

Mitral Valve Prolapse. The cause of chest pain in mitral valve prolapse, a familial syndrome with autosomal dominance, that occurs in approximately 5% of the population with a preponderance in females, is uncertain. When pain is present, it tends to be intermittent, apical, or epigastric, and is described as one of pressure. Bony anomalies, such as scoliosis, may also be present, and a recent study suggests that its incidence is higher in girls with anorexia nervosa and panic attacks. Auscultation reveals a nonejection, midsystolic click followed by a late systolic murmur. Diagnosis is confirmed by echocardiography.

Aortic Stenosis. Severe aortic stenosis or hypertrophic subaortic stenosis may be associated with epigastric or chest pain that is angina-like and worsened by effort. Although these lesions are usually diagnosed in early infancy, in some patients the diagnosis may not be made until adolescence. Sudden death in athletes with this condition has been reported, underscoring the necessity for auscultation of the heart as part of the pre-sports participation physical examination (see p. 172), and for taking seriously the history of exercise-associated dizziness or syncope.

Pulmonary Causes

In the adolescent with sudden onset of pain in the chest, a pulmonary cause is likely. The pain is typically well-localized and worsened by respiration. These patients look acutely ill and anxious, are dyspneic, and invariably have alterations in vital signs.

Pulmonary Embolism. Because this condition is rare in adolescents, it is often associated with delay in recognition and resulting death when it does occur. Predisposing conditions include obesity, postoperative state, chronic illness (such as sickle cell anemia) and, rarely, use of estrogen-containing oral contraceptives. The sharp, excruciating pain is associated with tachypnea, tachycardia, hypotension, and often with rales and a pleural friction rub, and is worsened by inspiration. The patients sits upright and looks acutely anxious. The tender cords of thrombophlebitis may be palpated in the calf.

Pleurisy. The pain is sharp, worsened by inspiration, and localized to the site of the underlying consolidation. Adolescents with pleurisy typically have signs and symptoms of an associated pneumonia: dyspnea, cough, fever, rales, bronchial breath sounds, and/or pleural friction rub. Once fluid accumulates, however, pain may subside. Less commonly, the pain may be dull and may be referred to the back or shoulder. Rarely, it may be caused by tuberculosis, inflammatory diseases such as systemic lupus erythematosus, or metastatic intrathoracic malignancy.

Pneumothorax. In the adolescent, a pneumothorax may result from rupture of a cyst or emphysematous bleb, trauma to the thorax, or secondary to a foreign body. Asthma, weight-lifting, or self-induced vomiting may precipitate rupture of a bleb. Spontaneous pneumothorax, without any apparent underlying defect, is more common in adolescent males than in any other age group. The sudden, sharp pain is typically accompanied by dyspnea and cyanosis. Percussion results in a finding of tympany and decreased breath sounds over the affected side. The larynx and trachea may be shifted to the opposite side.

BREAST PAIN

Pain in the breast is a common finding in adolescents of both sexes, albeit for different reasons. In males, breast pain may be associated with gynecomastia and may be accompanied by the finding of tenderness on palpation. Anxiety about having breasts, often coupled with fear of cancer, usually prompts the visit to the physician and should be responded to with reassurance. In females, pain in the breast is typically cyclical, occurring most often at mid-cycle and with menses. Such pain can often be eliminated with oral contraceptives. Painful breast masses are usually cysts or fibroadenomas, the former characteristically undergoing involution with subsequent menstrual cycles. As in male adolescents, fear of cancer is common among females with breast pain or a breast mass.

MUSCULOSKELETAL PAIN

Now referred to as the chest wall syndrome, the finding of pain, exacerbated by movement of the trunk and present at rest, and anterior chest wall tenderness with or without swelling at the costochondral junction, suggests that the problem is musculoskeletal in etiology. It includes other terms such as costochondritis, Tietze syndrome, and xiphodynia. This syndrome has been identified as the cause of chest pain in between 22 and 80% of adolescents with chest pain in various studies published in the past decade, suggesting that it is an important consideration in the differential diagnosis of this symptom. Response to nonsteroidal anti-inflammatory drugs is dramatic.

GASTROINTESTINAL PAIN

Esophagitis. Burning pain over the lower sternum and/or epigastrium suggests the possibility of esophageal dysfunction, the most common manifestation of which is esophagitis. The pain is substernal, gradual in onset, and intermittent, and is often accompanied by a bitter or sour taste. It is worsened by lying down, bending over, and meals, and rarely radiates to the back. The pain may be relieved by antacids. In adolescents, esophagitis or gastritis may result from ingestion of alcohol, recurrent vomiting (self-induced or spontaneous) or, in the case of the athlete, nonsteroidal anti-inflammatory agents.

Esophageal Tear. Rupture or tear of the esophagus is a rare occurrence but the seriousness of sequelae warrants its inclusion in this discussion. Self-induced vomiting, such as occurs in adolescent eating disorders, may be responsible. The pain is sudden and burning and is localized to the substernum or radiates to the neck. If the tear is above the gastroesophageal junction, pneumomediastinum may result, and crepitus, coordinated with cardiac contraction, is the primary finding on physical examination. If presence of an esophageal tear is suspected, appropriate contrast studies must be performed to establish the diagnosis and effect immediate surgical repair.

Psychogenic Causes

Chest pain of any origin in an adolescent may cause anxiety and be associated with negative life events. Regardless of etiology, reassurance and supportive therapy are as important as specific therapeutic interventions. The designation of pain as psychogenic is misleading, and is used in this discussion to describe chest pain not caused by structural or physiologic dysfunction. As will be seen, however, these conditions may, themselves, produce organic dysfunction.

Hyperventilation. Hyperventilation may be associated with transient, sharp pain in the left anterior precordial area that may be worsened by movement or deep inspiration. The pain is thought to be secondary to distention of the stomach that results from swallowing large amounts of air (aerophagia). Alternatively, it may be due to spasm of the left hemidiaphragm or secondary to the hypocapneic alkalosis of hyperventilation.

Idiopathic. When no organic cause is found, chest pain is referred to as idiopathic. In such cases, the pain is as real to the patient as it is in those in whom an organic explanation is found. The pain should be acknowledged and the patient instructed about techniques for self-mastery of pain, while offering reassurance that the pain is not due to cancer or a heart attack. Exploration about sources of stress should continue as the patient is followed. Somatic complaints may result from lack of appropriate counseling following rape or incest or any other traumatic event. Somatization disorders may also present with a complaint of pain.

Evaluation of the Adolescent with Short Stature

The tremendous range in normal heights and in timing of onset of the growth spurt, and the common concern among adolescents who are in any way different from their peers, combine to make stature an important issue, particularly among males. The role of the physician in evaluating the adolescent with short stature is to address the following questions:

1. Is the short stature a normal variant or the symptom of a pathologic process?
2. Regardless of etiology, is the adolescent experiencing psychological stress because of his or her height?
3. Is the adolescent a candidate for hormonal intervention?

NORMAL VARIANT OR PATHOLOGIC PROCESS?

The differential diagnosis of short stature includes a number of chromosomal, endocrine, skeletal, and chronic illnesses. Because most of these will present in infancy or childhood, this discussion focuses only on conditions that are likely to become apparent during adolescence (Table 31), recognizing that the others will continue to be associated with short stature in the adolescent years.

Constitutional Short Stature/Pubertal Delay

History. There is often a history of delay in growth in one or both parents during their adolescence. Of normal size at birth and throughout infancy, these patients typically begin to fall from their original percentile curve in the preschool years. After that, growth is steady at approximately 4

TABLE 31. Causes of Short Stature in an Adolescent Male

Familial
Constitutional delayed puberty
Endocrinopathies
Hypopituitarism (e.g., craniopharyngioma, glioma, trauma)
Cushing syndrome
Adrenal insufficiency
Diabetes mellitus (poorly controlled)
Chronic systemic illness
Gastrointestinal (e.g., Crohn disease)
Pulmonary (e.g., cystic fibrosis)
Renal (e.g., insufficiency)
Cardiac (cyanotic)
Undernutrition (e.g., anorexia nervosa)
Secondary to chronic illness
Secondary to depression
Anorexia nervosa

cm/yr, albeit at or below the 3rd percentile. There is absence of a history of headaches, visual disturbance, or abnormality in smell perception.

Physical Examination. Absence of signs of puberty by the age of 14.5 years is the accepted definition of pubertal delay in males and typically accompanies short stature. Physical examination is otherwise normal (that is, no abnormality in body proportions, thyroid function, or visual fields).

Laboratory Findings. A delayed bone age of more than 2 years is characteristic.

Follow-up. The patient should be reevaluated at 6-month intervals and reassured that the long period of slow growth with epiphyses still open will result in greater height than if puberty had been earlier, often sufficient consolation for having to wait. Use of testosterone in males over 14.5 years should be considered (see p. 128).

Acquired Hypopituitarism

History. The history will vary depending on the cause. Most cases of hypopituitarism that present during adolescence result from a neoplasm, the most common of which is craniopharyngioma and, less commonly, glioma. Accordingly, symptoms of headaches, visual disturbance, polydipsia, polyuria, or polyphagia may be found; however, more often, it is failure to develop secondary sex characteristics or experience the growth spurt at the age-appropriate time that causes an adolescent boy to present for evaluation.

Physical Examination. Signs of a neoplasm of the hypothalamic-pituitary axis, such as a visual field defect, may be found and there may be signs of increased intracranial pressure, such as papilledema. In many instances, however, the only physical finding is the lack of development of secondary sex characteristics.

Laboratory Evaluation. *Radiographic.* A calcified craniopharyngioma may be detected on lateral skull x-ray. Often, however, it is necessary to obtain a CT scan or MRI in order to demonstrate the presence of a tumor.

Growth Hormone. Deficiency of growth hormone may be an isolated finding or combined with deficiencies of other hormones produced by the pituitary gland. In this condition the level of growth hormones in the serum is low in multiple samples (see Appendix 8 for normal values) and does not show the expected rise after stimulation by exercise, insulin, arginine, glucagon, levodopa, or clonidine. An elevated growth hormone level is characteristic of anorexia nervosa.

LH, FSH, TSH (T4/T3), ACTH, and Vasopressin. Serum levels of these hormones may also be low. In females in whom gonadal dysgenesis is the cause of short stature, however, LH and FSH levels are extremely high. In the evaluation for possible thyroid dysfunction, it would be appropriate first to obtain a T4 level. Should this value be low, TSH would then be measured to ascertain whether the hypothyroidism is primary or secondary.

Other Endocrinopathies

Adrenal insufficiency, Cushing disease, or poorly controlled diabetes mellitus may be associated with short stature.

Chronic Systemic Illness

Any disease that impairs nutrition (such as Crohn disease or cystic fibrosis), decreases tissue oxygenation (such as cyanotic congenital heart disease or pulmonary disease), or causes renal insufficiency may be responsible for short stature if pubertal growth has not been completed at the time of onset.

Laboratory Evaluation. The following tests should be carried out to evaluate short stature in the adolescent with chronic illness:

Complete blood count (to rule out anemia, occult infection, or malignancy).

Erythrocyte sedimentation rate (ESR) (a good screening test for inflammatory bowel disease, infection, and malignancy, if elevated). A low ESR is found in anorexia nervosa.

Urinalysis (for renal dysfunction or infection).

Stool for ova, parasites, or occult blood (inflammatory bowel disease).

Blood urea nitrogen (renal dysfunction).

Serum sodium, potassium, chloride, bicarbonate (adrenal insufficiency, renal tubular dysfunction, and anorexia nervosa with bulimic features).

Undernutrition

Although anorexia nervosa is more common in young adolescent females, it also occurs in males. If its onset antedates that of the pubertal growth spurt, short stature may be a manifestation. Accordingly, a careful history of eating habits, possible distortion of body image, exercise, and purging should be obtained.

IS THE ADOLESCENT STRESSED BY SHORT STATURE?

Regardless of its cause, it is important to recognize that short stature may result in psychosocial stress in our culture, particularly for adolescent males. Studies have shown that delay in pubertal development is often associated with poorer school performance, poor self-image, and depression in males. The proper evaluation of the patient who presents with short stature includes screening for these areas of dysfunction. Intervention will vary with the findings and may range from counseling of parents who may have unrealistic athletic expectations of their late-developing son to psychiatric therapy, as necessary.

IS TREATMENT FOR SHORT STATURE INDICATED?

Identification and remediation of specific causes of short stature are likely to result in improved growth. When the diagnosis is familial short stature or constitutional delay in puberty, the question often arises as to whether hormonal intervention is indicated. At the time of this writing, it is not considered appropriate to treat such patients with growth hormone. The other option is treatment with testosterone. Because testosterone has been shown to be effective and safe and is not associated with diminution of ultimate height, the following questions will assist in evaluating its use for short stature:

1. Does the patient show evidence of poor self-image, social withdrawal, and/or depression that he attributes to his small size?
2. Is he 14 years of age or older without onset of secondary sex characteristics (SMR 1) or evidence of a growth spurt?
3. Is his serum testosterone level less than 100 ng/dl?

If the answer to #1 and 2 or 3 is yes, it is appropriate to administer depot testosterone, 100 mg IM once monthly for 4 months.

Evaluation of the Adolescent for Eating Disorders

Not only have eating disorders become more common in this society, which values thinness, but the publicity surrounding them has caused parents and physicians to mistake symptoms of other conditions for those of anorexia nervosa or bulima. The role of the primary care physician is:

1. Prevention
2. Early recognition
3. Differential diagnosis
4. Prevention and treatment of medical complications
5. *Not* psychiatric treatment!

The focus of this section is on the differential diagnosis of eating disorders, and on the ongoing evaluation of the patient diagnosed as having either anorexia nervosa or bulimia (Table 32). (Because most patients with these disorders are females, the patient is referred to as "she" in this discussion.)

ANOREXIA NERVOSA

The DSM III-R criteria for anorexia nervosa are listed in Table 33.

Criteria

Age: Between 10 and 40 years with onset of illness between 10 and 30 years. These age criteria are rather arbitrary and should be viewed as a reflection of the past experience with anorexia nervosa rather than as exclusion criteria. For example, we have seen patients present before the

TABLE 32. Differential Diagnosis of Anorexia Nervosa

Organic Disease
Endocrine
Diabetes mellitus
Hyperthyroidism
Neurologic
CNS neoplasm
Gastrointestinal
Inflammatory bowel disease
Achalasia
Neoplastic
Any malignancy
Gynecologic
Pregnancy
Immunologic
Lupus erythematosus
Psychiatric Disease
Depression
Thought disorder
Substance abuse

age of 10 years, and other investigators[65] have reported onset after the age of 60 years in a few patients.

Weight loss: Loss of at least 15% of original body weight and/or 15% below normal weight for age and height. The DSM III-R criteria use as their reference for these measurements the Metropolitan Life Insurance Policy Scales and the Iowa Growth Charts for Children. The experience that the former may present overly high figures for normal weights and that the latter are now outdated and based on a narrow ethnic segment of the population of the U.S. suggests that it may be more appropriate to use the data from the National Health Examination Survey (1966–1970), although

TABLE 33. DSM III-R Criteria for Anorexia Nervosa

1. Intense fear of becoming obese that does not diminish as weight loss progresses.
2. Disturbance in the way in which one's body weight, size, or shape is experienced: e.g., claiming to "feel fat" even when emaciated, or believing that one area of the body is "too fat" even when obviously underweight.
3. Refusal to maintain body weight over a minimal normal weight for age and height: e.g., weight loss leading to maintenance of body weight 15% below expected; failure to make expected weight gain during period of growth, leading to body weight 15% below expected.
4. In females, absence of at least three consecutive menstrual cycles when otherwise expected to occur (primary or secondary amenorrhea).

From Diagnostic and Statistical Manual of Mental Disorders III-R. Washington, DC, American Psychiatric Association, 1987, with permission.

these may also be approaching obsolescence. The recent addition of the consideration of lack of age-appropriate weight gain is an important factor for physicians caring for adolescent patients. The patient who fails to have a height and/or weight spurt by the age-appropriate time, or who fails to enter puberty or experience the timely progression of pubertal events, may have anorexia nervosa even if she has not actually lost 15% of body weight. It is important to note that when other criteria are present, the fact that weight loss has been less than that required by these criteria should not rule out the diagnosis. Because prognosis is better the earlier treatment is begun, a diagnosis should not await attainment of an arbitrary weight criterion.

Attitude Toward Weight and Food: Demonstration of a distorted attitude and behavior toward eating food or weight represented by any of the following:

Denial of illness with failure to recognize nutritional needs. Patients with anorexia nervosa not only deny that they are ill, but deny symptoms of hunger or any other symptoms (such as a cold). They also often rationalize their meager diets as being nutritionally sound and healthy. To this end, they rarely eat red meat and are often vegetarians, buying food at health food stores. Although they assiduously avoid fat or sugar-containing foods, they are likely to eat food high in protein (such as no-fat yogurt), albeit in very small amounts. They distort the caloric content of their food by greatly exaggerating it.

Apparent enjoyment of losing weight. They never get to a weight at which they feel they are thin, always being able to point to some part of their body, usually the thighs, that they demonstrate to be too fat by pinching some skin between the thumb and forefinger. The only exception is the patient who has read about the disease and recognizes that this is one of the bases for a diagnosis of anorexia nervosa and fears hospitalization if she admits to it. Such a patient may say that she realizes she is too thin and should gain weight. A provocative test for such a patient is instructing her to gain 1 pound within the week before she returns. This prescription is typically met with an immediate argument, a look of panic, or, more often, by weight loss by the next appointment and expressions of surprise.

Body image: A desired body image of extreme thinness. Hilda Bruch referred to this symptom as "relentless pursuit of thinness." In contrast to patients who have lost weight secondary to depression or organic illness, in whom its gradual nature remained unnoticed until it was extreme, those with anorexia nervosa can usually tell you the exact date their dieting and weight loss began (and occasionally its precipitant).

Eating habits. Unusual hoarding or handling of food. Rituals develop around food preparation or eating itself. Common among these is the process of cutting a piece of food into halves, then quarters, eighths, etc., and then eating only the last piece cut while believing to be eating it all. It is a useful diagnostic maneuver to arrange to meet the patient in the hospital cafeteria for lunch during the course of the initial visit to observe the youngster's eating behavior. This is often diagnostic!

At Least One of the Following Manifestations:

1. *Lanugo hair* (downy peige). A fine, hairy covering can be seen over the abdomen, back, and chest of severely malnourished patients with anorexia nervosa. The reason for its appearance is not known, but it has been postulated that it serves an insulating function in these patients, who are usually hypothermic (see below). Although patients rarely voluntarily inquire about lanugo hair, they are often relieved when it is acknowledged and they are told that it is reversible with nutritional rehabilitation.

2. *Bradycardia* (persistent resting pulse rate of 60 beats/min or less). Pulse rates may be as low as 22/min in our experience. Extreme bradycardia places patients with anorexia nervosa at high risk for superimposed ventricular arrhythmias, which may prove fatal. The reason for the bradycardia is speculative. Deficiency in production of norepinephrine/epinephrine, hypothalamic dysregulation, and the body's attempt to conserve energy have all been postulated mechanisms. In our experience, slowing of the pulse tends to follow lowering of body temperature; conversely, the pulse speeds up slightly when the patient is warmed above 36.2°C.

3. *Hypothermia* (temperature below 36.1°C). Patients with anorexia nervosa experience hypothermia as low as 33°C. This phenomenon is particularly striking when monitored during the night, and typically precedes bradycardia. The temperature should be confirmed with a rectal thermometer to ensure that core, rather than peripheral, temperature is being recorded. Reliance on oral temperature should be avoided, as patients frequently learn to drink warm water before their temperature is taken to avoid being hospitalized when extreme hypothermia is discovered. Many patients with anorexia nervosa who have contracted with their behavioral therapist for a certain weight gain each day learn (often from other patients) that they may do so without having to consume dreaded calories merely by stopping at the water fountain before reporting for weigh-in. As a result, these patients' oral temperatures will be artificially lowered by the cold water they drink. It is of interest that patients with anorexia nervosa who have hypothermia typically deny feeling cold and, in fact, lack the usual physiologic responses to low temperature levels such as "goose-flesh," piloerection, and shivering. The mechanisms responsible for the hypothermia of anorexia nervosa are still poorly defined. It has been suggested that it results from the body's attempt to conserve energy, from lack of adequate production of neurotransmitters (norepinephrine and epinephrine), and from hypothalamic dysregulation, or is related to the low levels of thyroid hormone seen in this condition.

4. *Episodes of bulimia* (compulsive overeating). Criteria for bulimia nervosa (more fully described in the following section), which may be present or absent in patients with anorexia nervosa, relate to the occurrence

of eating binges. In patients with pure bulimia, the binges may consist of ingestion of thousands of calories in high carbohydrate foods. In the patient with anorexia nervosa, the intake may be only a few hundred calories, thought by the patient with distorted, exaggerated idea of her intake to be a "binge."

5. *Vomiting* (may be self-induced). Following a binge, the patient may induce vomiting in order to rid her body of the dreaded calories. Others with this disease may engage in purgative behaviors in anticipation of a future indiscretion. Early on, vomiting is induced with the use of a finger (look for calluses or bruises across the knuckles, the point at which the teeth come in contact with the inciting hand), with the back of a spoon handle or other inanimate objects, or with ipecac (the most dangerous method because of the risk of cardiac damage from emetine). After a few months, however, most patients find they can induce vomiting by auto-suggestion or Valsalva maneuver. Possible indicators of the presence of recurrent vomiting include erosion of tooth enamel (particularly noticeable on the lingual aspect of the dentition), subconjunctival hemorrhage, parotid gland enlargement, metabolic alkalosis (urinary pH typically above 7.5), and hypokalemia. Life-threatening complications such as esophageal tears or ruptures have also occurred in these patients. These patients may engage in surreptitious vomiting followed by bizarre and secretive hiding of their vomitus.

Periods of Overactivity. This criterion relates to the common finding of excessive physical activity for the purpose of expending unwanted calories. This behavior may follow a meal, or in some anxious patients may occur early in the morning so as to anticipate consumption of calories in the future. These patients may engage in organized sports at school, but often are also solitary runners or work out alone. They rarely sit still, even when placed at bed rest in the hospital. Whereas most patients with anorexia nervosa encountered in the past manifested this symptom, in our most recent experience a large number of patients with bulimia nervosa are sedentary yet have all other typical features, suggesting that this criterion may not be essential to the diagnosis.

Amenorrhea of at Least Three Months' Duration (unless illness occurs before onset of menses). Amenorrhea may therefore be either secondary or primary. Although this symptom is shared with other conditions of malnutrition, it differs from them in that it may antedate the onset of extreme weight loss by many months. In our patient population, one-third of patients experienced amenorrhea more than 8 months before significant weight loss had occurred. Moreover, more than half fail to experience return of normal menstrual function within 1 year of weight rehabilitation following therapy. In taking a history from a patient suspected of having anorexia nervosa, it is important to inquire specifically about possible use of oral contraceptives, as these will result in the appearance of normal menstruation. The fact that patients with anorexia nervosa are appearing at younger ages than previously has given rise to another finding related to primary amenorrhea—pubertal delay. In our experience, the delay may be more significant for secondary sex characteristics that result from stimulation of estrogen, rather than androgen, so that pubic hair development is less delayed than is breast development.

No Known Medical Illness That Could Account for the Anorexia and Weight Loss. This criterion serves as an important reminder to physicians to consider the entire differential diagnosis of these symptoms (Table 34) so as to exclude organic causes. Rarely, however, patients with organic illness may also develop anorexia nervosa.

No Other Major Psychiatric Disorder (such as major affective disorder or schizophrenia). Some of the symptoms of these conditions may be shared with anorexia nervosa but in psychiatric disorders, weight loss is usually a by-product, rather than the avowed goal, of their behavior. Similarly, the distortion of body image is missing in patients with these diagnoses.

Classifications

Patients with anorexia nervosa may be subdivided on the basis of psychological and behavioral characteristics. Such subclassification is useful in terms of psychological and medical management and serves to remind us that not all patients with anorexia nervosa are the same. Strober,[62] for example, has subtyped patients with anorexia nervosa on the basis of four factors:

Factor Analysis

Factor 1. Referred to by him as "the general anorexia symptom" factor, this was found to be associated with perfectionism and competitive athletic involvement.

Factor 2. This "mood" and "dysregulation" factor correlated with depression and family history of obesity, alcoholism, and depression.

Factor 3. Anxiety and compulsive-perfectionistic traits characterized this subgroup.

Factor 4. Patients in this group were found to be cognitively and developmentally immature.

Eating Behavior

Another common basis for classification of patients with anorexia nervosa relates to their eating behavior:

Restrictors. These patients achieve weight loss by strict control over the number of calories consumed. They also often engage in rigorous physical activity to burn up calories.

Anorectics with Bulimic Features. These patients may experience periodic episodes of binge eating, but their binges, in contrast to those of the true bulimics (below), typically consist of a few hundred, as opposed to a few thousand, calories. They are more likely than their restrictor counterparts to use laxatives or to self-induce vomiting and are less likely to engage in athletic activities.

Water Consumption

Our experience suggests that another useful basis for classification of patients with anorexia nervosa, in addition to the two described above, relates to attitudes about water consumption:

Water Restrictors. These patients' distorted body image has resulted in their feeling "fat" after drinking large amounts of water. Accordingly, they avoid water and often become dehydrated.

Water Loaders. These patients learn that they can achieve their contracted-for weight gain without consumption of dreaded calories by drinking large amounts of water. They may develop dilutional hyponatremia as a complication of this behavior.

Physical Evaluation

Every organ system in the body is affected by anorexia nervosa, so that a careful examination is required to appreciate the myriad of possible complications, as well as to prevent and recognize risk factors for death in this disease, which has a mortality rate of 10–15%. Moreover, the similarity between signs and symptoms of anorexia nervosa and a number of organic illnesses challenges even the most astute diagnostician.

General. Typically dressed in bulky, although stylish, clothing and meticulously groomed and made-up, her cheerful demeanor appears in marked contrast to the associated emaciation. Males, however, are characterized solely by the latter.

Vital signs.

Pulse: Typically less than 60/min.

Blood pressure: low with postural changes common

Temperature: less than 36.2°C, particularly if checked during the night or early morning hours.

HEENT. Hair loss is most likely to occur during the refeeding phase. Subconjunctival hemorrhage suggests the possibility of vomiting (although its absence does not eliminate this possibility). Disk margins are sharp (this is an important sign in differentiating anorexia nervosa from increased intracranial pressure secondary to a central nervous system neoplasm, which may also cause weight loss and amenorrhea). Teeth may show enamel erosion on the palatine surface if recurrent vomiting has occurred. The gag reflex may be absent in chronic self-induced vomiters and the pharynx may show lacerations as a result of use of sharp objects to induce vomiting. Tympanic membranes are retracted.

Neck. Parotid swelling may occur in patients with bulimic features. Presence of enlarged lymph nodes suggests the possibility of malignancy, rather than anorexia nervosa. Enlarged thyroid gland may signify either hyperthyroidism or hypothyroidism, either of which may share certain signs of anorexia nervosa (weight loss, amenorrhea or hypothermia, and bradycardia). Crepitus is a rare but potentially important sign of pneumomediastinum secondary to esophageal tear or rupture in the patient who vomits.

Breasts. Pubertal delay or interruption in development of the breasts is not uncommon. Hypoplasia of breasts may occur, depending on the time of onset.

Cardiac. In addition to extreme bradycardia, the finding of an arrhythmia is an indication for immediate hospitalization with cardiac monitoring. An arrhythmia is the most common cause of death in these patients. Signs of congestive failure may occur in the patient who suddenly overeats and drinks in order to avoid hospitalization. An increased association between anorexia nervosa and mitral valve prolapse has been reported.

Abdomen. The typical picture is that of a scaphoid abdomen with hard stool palpable within the colon. Palpation should serve to rule out other causes of amenorrhea and weight loss, such as an ovarian neoplasm or pregnancy.

Genitalia. Pubertal delay may be found by examination of pubic hair, although there is usually less retardation in this parameter than in that of breast development. Evidence of hypoestrogenism, another manifestation of anorexia nervosa, is apparent in examination of the vaginal mucosa, which will be thin, red, and dry. Because the differential diagnosis of amenorrhea includes masculinizing endocrinopathies, the size of the clitoris should be evaluated (see p. 84 and Appendix 7). The possibility of pregnancy should be ruled out by appropriate examination and laboratory testing. In males, pubertal delay also occurs, and testes may be soft or atrophic.

Musculoskeletal. An increased incidence of scoliosis in patients with anorexia nervosa has been reported (as has Turner syndrome). Turner syndrome should be considered in the patient with anorexia nervosa and short stature, particularly if other stigmata, such as webbed neck and widely spaced nipples, are noted. Osteoporosis, a common complication of hypoestrogenism, has no obvious physical findings (except if a stress fracture has occurred). Muscular weakness and tenderness may result from toxicity of emetine, the major ingredient in ipecac used to induce vomiting. (If this is suspected, the possibility of potentially fatal cardiac toxicity should be immediately investigated.) Muscle weakness is also a sign of hypokalemia, another complication of recurrent vomiting of any etiology or laxative use.

Skin. Dry skin and lanugo hair characterize patients with anorexia nervosa. Those who induce vomiting with their fingers may also have scars or lacerations across their knuckles.

Laboratory Evaluation

The following tests should be done to rule out other causes of weight loss and amenorrhea, as well as to evaluate the physiologic status of the patient with a confirmed diagnosis of anorexia nervosa, and thus guide management.

- Complete blood count: Patients with anorexia nervosa typically have neutropenia and may have iron deficiency anemia.
- Erythrocyte sedimentation rate (ESR). Low in anorexia nervosa (1–6 mm/hr); elevated in inflammatory bowel disease. The ESR may, however, be in the normal range in patients with inflammatory bowel disease who are extremely malnourished.
- Urinalysis: A high urinary pH suggests the possibility of purging, and pseudoproteinuria is commonly found when dipsticks are used on alkaline urines. Urine specific gravity may be very low in water loaders or high in water restrictors. Dehydrated patients often show pyuria and hematuria as well. Obviously, other causes for these findings should be sought (such as infection).
- Pregnancy test (preferably a beta subunit HCG serum test).
- CT scan of the head to rule out a central nervous system tumor.
- Serum levels of gonadotropins. FSH and LH are low in anorexia nervosa, elevated in gonadal dysfunction, and discordant in polycystic ovary syndrome (FSH = normal, LH 3× FSH).
- Serum level of prolactin: Normal or low in anorexia nervosa, elevated in many other causes of amenorrhea.
- Serum level of estradiol: Low in anorexia nervosa, sports amenorrhea.
- Serum level of progesterone: Low in the absence of ovulation of any etiology.
- T4 and T3 levels are usually low, with a normal TSH level and elevated reverse T3 in anorexia nervosa.
- Serum level of growth hormone: This is elevated although somatomedin C levels are low in anorexia nervosa.
- Cortisol levels are elevated without diurnal variation and fail to suppress with dexamethasone in anorexia nervosa.
- BUN may be elevated in dehydrated patients but this may be balanced by low protein intake.
- SGPT may be mildly elevated in starvation of any etiology.
- Potassium levels may be slightly low on the basis of decreased intake or markedly low secondary to purging.
- Bicarbonate levels are elevated in those who purge.

- Calcium and magnesium levels may be low in patients with malabsorption secondary to abuse of laxatives.
- Sodium may be low (dilutional) in water loaders.
- Zinc levels are low but not a reliable test in routine labs.
- Amylase levels may be elevated, particularly in those with bulimic features.
- Stool testing for phenolphthalein, an ingredient in many laxatives: This test is performed by alkalinization of liquid stool. Pink color indicates a positive test.
- Bone density may be low in those with severe malnutrition, prolonged amenorrhea or pubertal delay.
- ECG: Low voltage is common in anorexia nervosa, as is bradycardia; rarely, ST segment depression is found. A low t-wave is suggestive of hypokalemia, and a reversed t-wave may result from ipecac poisoning. A prolonged QTc (> 0.44 sec) and arrhythmias may also be found in patients with anorexia nervosa.

BULIMIA

Bulimia, from a Greek word meaning "ox hunger," refers to the occurrence of binge eating in a normal or overweight person. Although approximately half of adolescent patients with anorexia nervosa may have bulimic features to their illness either at presentation or at follow-up, it is now recognized that bulimia can exist as a separate entity. The DSM III-R criteria for bulimia are listed in Table 34.

Physical Examination

The physical examination may be normal, as these patients are typically of normal or above-normal weight. However, among those who purge, the method used for purging or complications of purging may lead to physical findings. The physical examination should serve to rule out any organic conditions that may be responsible for recurrent vomiting, such as inflamma-

TABLE 34. DSM III-R Criteria for Bulimia Nervosa

1. Recurrent episodes of binge eating (rapid consumption of a large amount of food in a discrete period of time, usually less than 2 hours.)
2. During the eating binges, a fear of not being able to stop eating.
3. Regularly engaging in self-induced vomiting, use of laxatives, or rigorous dieting or fasting in order to counteract the effects of binge eating.
4. A minimum average of two binge eating episodes per week for at least 3 months.

From Diagnostic and Statistical Manual of Mental Disorders III-R. Washington, DC, American Psychiatric Association, 1987, with permission.

tory bowel disease, achalasia, increased intracranial pressure, pancreatitis, or pregnancy. General appearance and vital signs are typically normal.

HEENT. Rule out increased intracranial pressure secondary to a CNS neoplasm by examination of the optic disks. Subconjunctival hemorrhage may be present in those who induce vomiting, although this is not a common finding. Palatine surface of teeth may show enamel erosion. The gag reflex may be absent and the pharynx may be lacerated.

Neck. Parotid swelling may occur secondary to binging or vomiting. Crepitus may result from pneumomediastinum secondary to esophageal tear (this is a medical emergency).

Cardiac. Irregular rhythm may suggest emetine poisoning secondary to ingestion of ipecac in large doses for the purpose of inducing vomiting.

Musculoskeletal. Weakness and aching of skeletal muscles are other manifestations of emetine toxicity. Muscle weakness may also result from hypokalemia secondary to purging.

Skin. Scars, calluses, or scratches on the dorsum of the knuckles may result from use of fingers to induce vomiting.

Laboratory Evaluation

- CT scan should be performed if any concern exists that vomiting may be secondary to increased intracranial pressure.
- Erythrocyte sedimentation rate (ESR) is elevated in patients whose vomiting is due to Crohn disease of the esophagus.
- Urinalysis: pH is elevated and pseudoproteinuria is found in recurrent vomiters, the latter when a urine dipstick is used.
- Pregnancy test is performed to rule out pregnancy as the cause of recurrent vomiting.
- Serum electrolytes: Low potassium and elevated bicarbonate secondary to vomiting and/or stool losses. Magnesium and calcium may be low in chronic abusers of laxatives.
- Amylase: Levels may be high secondary to binging and/or vomiting.
- Barium swallow should be performed if there is concern that recurrent vomiting may be secondary to achalasia (occasionally this may be seen on routine chest x-ray, which should therefore be taken first) or Crohn disease of the esophagus. Stool for phenolphthalein (see above).

OBESITY

Approximately 15% of adolescents are estimated to be obese. There has been a 40% increase in obesity among adolescents over the past 15 years in the U.S. The determinants of obesity are multiple and its prevalence varies with sex, socioeconomic and ethnic status, and familial factors. Among adolescents, obesity is more common in those from lower socioeconomic strata, in whites, and in native Americans.

Obesity refers to the condition of excess fat tissue. Operationalization of this term is variable because of the difficulty of accurately and practically measuring adipose tissue. Indirect measures are often used and have obvious methodologic limitations. Among them, the most common method is determination of skinfold thickness at three to seven standard sites of the body, including the subscapular, triceps, and suprailiac areas. The relationship between skinfold thickness and body fat is shown in Table 18. An adolescent may be considered to be obese if the skinfold thickness is greater than the 85th percentile for age and sex.

An alternative interpretation of the term obese is being more than 20% above what is considered desirable weight for height, sex, and age. Such a definition ignores the fact that tissues other than fat contribute to body weight and that the large-boned or very muscular adolescent may be at a higher weight for height than his similarly tall reference group and yet not have excess fat.

Developmental issues must also be considered. For boys, for example, there is a transient increase in body fat just before puberty, followed by a decrease as muscle tissue increases. For girls, puberty is associated with a steady increase in body fat, secondary to increasing estrogen levels, reaching approximately 25% for most at the completion of puberty. Longitudinal studies of adipocyte development suggest that individuals destined to be obese show a significant increase in fat cell size after the age of 17 years.

Although obesity during adulthood clearly shortens life expectancy by increasing the risk of life-threatening diseases, and despite the fact that obesity during adolescence predisposes to obesity during adulthood, obesity *per se* during childhood does not appear to present a health hazard. Because obesity is often associated with elevated cholesterol and triglyceride levels, and occasionally with high blood pressure, however, the obese adolescent should be evaluated for these possibilities. Obesity during adolescence may also predispose to stress of certain parts of the skeletal system, so that knee dysfunction and slipped capital femoral epiphysis are more common in the markedly obese. Another physical effect of obesity is acceleration of the pubertal process. In general, obese girls have an earlier onset of menses than those who are lean. Acceleration of puberty is also associated with an earlier growth spurt and resultant shorter ultimate height.

The most significant health-related problem of obese adolescents appears to be related to the psychosocial ramifications of growing up in a society that abhors and fears fatness. The self-esteem of middle-class obese adolescents appears to be lower than that of their normal-weight peers and they are more likely to suffer from depression. These findings may not be generalizable to all obese adolescents, however.

Genetic, metabolic, or endocrine causes of obesity are rare in adolescents (less than 2%). If obesity is associated with mental retardation and hypogonadism, Laurence-Moon-Beidl or Prader-Willi syndromes should be considered. If bone age and height are at or above average, hypothyroidism should not be considered. Most adolescent obesity can therefore be considered to be "exogenous," a term further subdivided by Mellin[38] to include psychologic, social, and behavioral factors. She defines "progressive" obesity as that which is related to the diet and exercise patterns within families and is manifested by steady weight gain throughout childhood. The other subcategory of exogenous adolescent obesity in Mellin's classification is "reactive" or, according to Bruch, "emotional" overeating. This refers to adolescents who are depressed or passive and who eat when under stress. As a result, their weight gain is episodic and they often engage in binge-eating. Mellin believes that the second subtype predominates in adolescence. Contrary to popular belief, however, it has been shown that obese adolescents do not typically eat more that their lean peers. What does appear to differentiate obese adolescents is their pattern of eating, which is very irregular and faster. Another important difference relates to physical activity, which is clearly less among obese adolescents. Television watching is greater among obese than normal-weight adolescents, and studies have shown that the prevalence of obesity increases by 2% for each hour of television watching.

Successful intervention strategies for weight reduction in obese adolescents have focused on diet control and exercise, improving self-esteem, and increasing self-efficacy to produce slow, steady weight loss of two pounds each week. Setting realistic goals for desirable weight loss and avoiding starvation diets, use of diuretics, appetite-suppressant drugs, laxatives, or self-induced vomiting are particularly important at this age. Unknown to most is the fact that a starvation diet may be perfectly adequate for adults, but adolescents require between 2500 (females) and 3000 (males) calories to support pubertal growth. They also must ensure an adequate intake of vitamins and mineral to fuel this growth spurt. In order for a weight-reduction program to be successful, however, the adolescent must be motivated. Forcing an unmotivated teenager into a weight loss program will serve only to increase his or her sense of failure. Programs that include peer support and behavior modification techniques are the most successful.

Evaluation of Compliance in the Adolescent Patient

The extent of noncompliance among adolescent patients is no different from that in adults, but its determinants and consequences are sufficiently unique to deserve special consideration. The possibility of noncompliance is usually first raised when a patient does not improve. Particularly when treating adolescent patients, however, it is important that such a situation be prevented, lest the adolescent be allowed to fail in what is often his or her first independent experience as a patient. It is necessary to be able to identify the teenager who is at risk for noncompliance before it occurs, so that there can be closer monitoring and support offered. The Adolescent Compliance Prediction Checklist is a useful instrument for this task (Table 35). A score of less than 5 portends poor compliance; between 6 and 12, compliance may be problematic; and 13 or above, the risk of noncompliance is small. The list is derived from the literature on compliance, as well as from our own experience in prospective evaluation of adolescent patients in a variety of clinical situations. It has been shown to be useful for adolescents required to take long-term medication for a chronic illness or for contraception, as well as for those requested to return for medical appointments. Factors to be considered in the evaluation of the adolescent patient include:

What Are the Patient's Health Beliefs?

Work by Becker et al.[3] has demonstrated that the patient's belief about his or her illness, the efficacy of the proposed treatment, and the competency of the physician are more important in determining compliance than is the reality of the situation. Patients from cultures other than the prevailing one in this country may have special health beliefs that will influence their

TABLE 35. Adolescent Compliance Prediction Checklist

I. Data Base (General)
 A. Health Beliefs (patient's perception of the following)
  1. Susceptibility ______
  2. Seriousness of illness ______
  3. Belief in efficacy of treatment ______
 B. "Reality" Factors
  1. Experience with the disease:
   a. Length of time ______
   b. Complications ______
   c. Others with the disease (family, friends) ______
  2. Experience with the medication:
   a. Side effects in past ______
   b. Difficulty remembering (this vs. other meds) ______
   c. Knowledge of side effects in friends or relatives with this medication
   ______
  3. Experience with the therapist/setting:
   a. "Satisfied" ______
   b. Problems ______
 C. Developmental Factors
  1. Age
  2. Tanner stage
  (1–2) → Early vs. late maturer? ______
  3. Autonomy—setting appointments, job, school, choice of friends, etc.
  ______
 D. Psychosocial Factors (using standardized instruments)
  1. Self-image ______
  2. Conflict with family ______
  3. "Self-reliance" ______
  4. "Personal freedom" ______

willingness to comply with prescribed treatment. It is important that the physician encourage that these beliefs be aired and respected and that attempts be made to reconcile them with the proposed therapy.

What Is the Reality of the Patient's Medical Status?

In addition to the patient's beliefs about his or her health, the actual experience with the illness and the health care system appears to be an important determinant of future compliance. For example, it has been shown that a patient who has experienced a condition previously, or who has had a close relationship with someone who has, is likely to be more compliant than one who has just contracted it. With adolescents, however, the impact of such experience will vary with the patient's stage of cognitive and psychosocial development (see below Developmental Factors). As with adult patients, compliance among adolescents appears better when the condition has not persisted for more than 6 months.

What Is the Patient's Stage of Development?

The adolescent patient's maturity, both physical and psychosocial, appears to have a tremendous effect on willingness and ability to comply with the recommendations of the health care provider. Accordingly, if he or she feels invulnerable, knowledge that another patient had dire consequences from noncompliance will have little bearing on compliance. In a healthy, sexually active patient for whom oral contraceptives have been prescribed, her worry that she may be unable to become pregnant may be a potent determinant of noncompliance, despite the doctor's concern about risk of pregnancy. Similarly, an adolescent who is sexually active but not yet able to think abstractly will have difficulty internalizing the notion that she is at risk for pregnancy. Our studies have shown that the adolescent with a positive self-image (measured by the Piers-Harris Self-Concept Scale) and who is acting in an autonomous manner (i.e., making own appointments with the doctor, setting the agenda for the medical visit, filling the prescription, and/or scoring high in standardized tests of autonomy such as the California Test of Personality subscale can be expected to comply with the prescription and with appointment-keeping. Conversely, depression, not surprisingly, is associated with poor compliance, not only with medications and appointment-keeping, but also with use of automotive safety devices such as seat belts and helmets.

One may question the absence from the evaluation of the issue of knowledge about the disease or medication. It has been well demonstrated that knowledge is a necessary prerequisite to compliance but it alone is not sufficient to ensure it. Similarly, frightening the adolescent patient about the consequences of noncompliance has been shown to be counterproductive and may actually promote noncompliance.

Evaluation of the Adolescent Patient for Contraception

Once it is determined that the adolescent patient is sexually active (see pp. 21–27 for guidelines for taking a sexual history), he or she must be evaluated to determine the level of motivation and the best method of contraception to be recommended. Table 36 lists the issues to be considered in the evaluation, which are discussed below.

AGE

Physicians are often reluctant to prescribe hormonal contraception (specifically, estrogen) for young adolescent females, fearing that growth may be compromised. There is now ample evidence, however, that the small amount of estrogen in birth control pills (35 or 50 μg) is insufficient for causing closure of epiphyses. Moreover, by the time most adolescents present for birth control, they have already passed the peak of their growth velocity curve (see p. 45). There is also concern that starting an adolescent female on hormonal contraception commits her to what may be a dangerously long period of use with possible later consequences. Although this may be theoretically correct, there are presently no supportive data. A more common problem is cessation of use after months, not years, of use. Age has an indirect effect on some of the other issues to be considered in that the younger the patient, the less likely it is that her parents know about her sexual activity, the less likely she is to have a supportive partner, and the less likely she is to be able to think abstractly in terms of the risk for becoming pregnant.

TABLE 36. Issues To Be Considered in Evaluating An Adolescent for Contraception

Age
Frequency of intercourse
Past experience with contraceptives
Attitude of friends/partner about contraception/ methods
Knowledge and attitudes of parents
Medical history
Family history
Comfort with body
Cultural attitudes
Risk of sexually transmitted disease
Vulnerability/motivation
Potential for compliance

FREQUENCY OF INTERCOURSE

It has been our experience that the more frequent the intercourse, the more likely it is that the adolescent will acknowledge to herself that she is sexually active, and the more likely she is to obtain contraception and be compliant with it. Conversely, infrequent intercourse is associated with poorer compliance and with the tendency for each episode to be rationalized as unexpected. The method of contraception suitable for each extreme of the frequency distribution may also be different. Frequent intercourse necessitates continuous protection that might be achieved by daily use of oral contraceptives or injectable progestin. When intercourse is infrequent, however, consideration may be given to a diaphragm, condom, and foam, or "morning after" pill (for example, Ovral given in a dose of two pills immediately upon discovery of unprotected intercourse within the prior 72 hours followed by another two pills 12 hours thereafter).

PAST EXPERIENCE WITH CONTRACEPTIVES

A patient who has experienced side effects from a contraceptive agent in the past or who has had difficulty with compliance is likely to reject or discontinue use when it is prescribed again. If a pill of a different composition is chosen, it is important that the differences be stressed, lest the patient believe that all contraceptive pills are alike. Vicarious or heresay negative experiences (such as from a friend or from something read in the newspaper) may be equally predictive of failure if they have led the patient to think of the prescribed contraceptive as being harmful.

ATTITUDES OF OTHERS

When friends or, more importantly, the sexual partner speaks negatively about one or another contraceptive method, it is unlikely that it will be accepted and used. It is important that the partner be included in the discussion whenever possible and that the patient be asked to indicate any negative information she has received about the method under consideration.

PARENTS

In our experience, approximately half of the teenagers we see have told their parents about their sexual activity, albeit under a variety of circumstances. For those who feel that they cannot discuss the issue with their parents, choice of a contraceptive method must take into consideration their need for confidentiality. Thus, a diaphragm or pill compact may be problematic for the young girl whose mother may search her purse, whereas a prefilled applicator of spermicidal foam packaged to resemble a tampon may go unnoticed. An intrauterine device (IUD) or injectable progestin also has the advantage of being undetectable.

MEDICAL HISTORY

A careful medical history is mandatory to exclude any potential contraindications to use of one or another method of contraception. The first of these is a history of salpingitis, which is a contraindication for use of an IUD because of the increased risk of salpingitis and subsequent infertility in adolescents who use IUDs. It is useful to know if the patient has been pregnant in the past, as a positive history makes her a better candidate for an IUD. On the other hand, having become pregnant while using one contraceptive method surely indicates the need to try another. The adolescent female who has become pregnant while using contraception or who has been noncompliant may be considered a good candidate for injectable medroxyprogesterone (Depo-Provera) or implantable norgestrel (Norplant) when these agents are released for use. A history of toxic shock syndrome (TSS) should be a signal for caution in recommending any method that remains in the vaginal vault for more than 6 hours, such as a diaphragm, cervical cap, or contraceptive "sponge," as these agents have all been implicated in the pathogenesis of TSS and may increase the risk of its recurrence.

Having a chronic illness places the adolescent patient at increased risk for certain complications of contraceptive use. For example, estrogens are contraindicated in patients with sickle cell disease, liver disease, replaced cardiac valves, migraine headaches, lupus erythematosus, cystic fibrosis, or a history of thrombophlebitis. Diabetes mellitus is considered to be a relative contraindication to the use of estrogen-containing oral contraceptives. Hypertension is also a relative contraindication to use of either estrogen or progestin, and a cautious trial is suggested in order to determine if a given patient reacts adversely to either. The all-progestin pill is a reasonable alternative to that which contains a combination of estrogen and progestin for such patients if they desire to use an oral contraceptive. Although there have been no reports, thus far, of myocardial infarction or cerebrovascular accidents among adolescent smokers, the significantly increased risk for these complications among women over the age of 35 years who both smoke and use estrogen-containing oral contraceptives suggests that caution be used in prescribing these agents to adolescents who smoke more than one pack of cigarettes daily. Mental retardation is another important factor in choosing a birth control method. Adolescent females who are retarded are not only unable to attend to the need to use a contraceptive method but are often poorly able to care for their own hygienic needs and also may be at increased risk for sexual abuse. For all of these reasons, they are excellent candidates for injectable progestin (medroxyprogesterone, Depo-Provera).

FAMILY HISTORY

A family history of migraine or thrombophlebitis should be regarded as a relative contraindication to the use of estrogen-containing oral contraceptives.

COMFORT WITH ONE'S BODY

The teenager who expresses reluctance or disgust at the mention of inserting a tampon is unlikely to be a suitable candidate for use of any contraceptive method that requires touching the genitals, such as a diaphragm, cervical cap, spermicidal foam, jelly, or cream, or even an IUD.

CULTURAL ATTITUDES

In certain cultures and religious groups, use of any method of contraception, other than abstinence, is forbidden. It is obviously necessary for the physician treating the sexually active adolescent to know his or her beliefs about birth control and to try to take these into consideration.

RISK OF SEXUALLY TRANSMITTED DISEASE

Because adolescents have the highest rate of sexually transmitted diseases of any age group, choice of a contraceptive method should consider prevention of infection. The combination of a condom and spermicidal foam provides the best protection against infections and also provides acceptable protection against pregnancy when used by both partners. Their use should therefore be encouraged for teenagers with multiple sexual partners or otherwise at high risk for infection, recognizing that such partners are unlikely to comply. Conversely, methods such as the combination oral contraceptive pill, which is very effective for preventing pregnancy, does nothing to protect against venereal disease.

MOTIVATION

The adolescent who believes that he or she is unable to impregnate or conceive is not able to respond appropriately to the physician's admonitions about the risk of pregnancy. Some teenagers fear sterility as a result of having had the experience of intercourse without becoming pregnant. Alternatively, a teenager who has had a sexually transmitted disease may worry that it has caused sterility, despite adequate treatment. It is important for the physician to encourage expression of such concerns, should they exist, in order to provide reassurance and motivation for using birth control.

POTENTIAL FOR COMPLIANCE

Teenage patients who have had difficulty completing a course of any medication previously prescribed are unlikely to be good candidates for oral contraceptives, which require daily administration. As indicated above, a history of noncompliance with a contraceptive method portends failure should it be again prescribed. The adolescent with poor self-image and who is not acting autonomously is at high risk for noncompliance and for pregnancy.

Evaluation of the Adolescent Who Has Been Raped

Between one-quarter and one-half of rape victims in the U.S. are adolescents. Approximately 10% are males. The impact of this crime of violence on the adolescent may differ significantly from that in the younger child or adult, depending on the victim's stage of psychosocial development. The role of the primary care physician in the evaluation of the adolescent rape victim is *not* to establish validity of the claim of rape, but rather to proceed in a sensitive and supportive manner to accomplish the following tasks:

1. To treat any physical injuries
2. To collect evidence for legal prosecution
3. To prevent sexually transmitted diseases
4. To prevent pregnancy
5. To prevent psychological sequelae

PHYSICAL INJURIES

Approximately 50% of female adolescent rape victims manifest physical evidence of forcible intercourse. Severe vaginal and vaginoperineal lacerations are less common in this age group than in younger children. Among male victims, however, the incidence of serious anal laceration and/or hematoma is significant. More common than genital, anal, or perineal injuries, however, are injuries of other areas of the body sustained in the course of coercion, which may be serious and even fatal. The evaluation of the adolescent rape victim must include careful inspection of the entire body, even if he or she does not recall having sustained such injuries. If there is no external evidence of bleeding or trauma, a speculum examination is

TABLE 37. Physical Examination of the Adolescent Rape Victim

1. Vital signs
2. Emotional Status: The patient's own words should be used without editorializing or making legal judgments (see below)
3. General Appearance: Include notation about the condition of clothing
4. Body Surface: Locate and describe in words, as well as on a drawing, any injuries (e.g., ligature marks, abrasions, ecchymoses, bite marks, open wounds)
5. Mouth
6. Fingernails: Note if broken and collect scrapings
7. External Genitalia: Note injuries, presence of blood, and state of the hymen
8. Pelvic Examination: This examination is indicated if history and/or inspection of the external genitalia or rectum suggests penetration. The specimens needed for prosecution can be obtained without a speculum examination (see Table 38)

usually not indicated. A checklist for the physical examination of the rape victim is provided in Table 37.

COLLECTION OF MEDICOLEGAL EVIDENCE

Even if the rape victim indicates unwillingness to press charges, every effort should be made to collect the evidence needed for prosecution in the event that he or she later decides to do so. The specifics of evidence collection vary among the states, and local law enforcement agencies should be contacted to be sure that the examining physician is in compliance with local statutes. Collected specimens must be kept in the physical possession of the physician and signed over to the police at the appropriate time ("preserving the chain of custody"). The physician should avoid using language in the medical record that might unfairly influence a jury, such as statements to the effect that the patient "did not appear upset" (recalling that everyone has different coping mechanisms) or that she "alleges" to have been raped. A typical example of materials needed for evidence in a case of rape is presented in Table 38. The following should be obtained as evidence:

Clothing. Stained and/or torn clothing should be placed in a paper bag, sealed, and labeled.

Fingernail Scrapings. If the history suggests any attempt on the part of the victim to scratch the assailant, material (skin, hair, dirt, etc.) under the fingernails may assist in identification of the assailant. This material should be scraped from the underside of the nails with a wooden applicator (orange) stick or fingernail clipper. The material from each hand should be placed in a separate and appropriately labeled specimen vial.

Pubic and Other Body Hair. Retrieve and preserve any loose foreign hairs found during inspection of the body. In addition, pluck (do not cut) and separately save and label, in two envelopes, three pubic hairs from the patient's right and left side. Do the same with three hairs from each side of

TABLE 38. Collection of Evidence (and Useful Laboratory Tests) in a Case of Rape*

Clothing
Fingernail scrapings
Pubic and other body hair
Wood lamp examination
Sperm motility
Saline wash and dry specimens for spermatozoa
Acid phosphatase
Stool guaiac
Dipstick for occult blood in urine
VDRL
Pregnancy test
Cultures for gonococcus and chlamydia

*A kit containing the necessary swabs, vials, etc., as well as a checklist to document that each of these has been performed, made up in advance, is useful for the smooth conduct of the evaluation.

the patient's head. This aspect of specimen collection may be done at a later time by the criminology staff.

Wood Lamp Examination. Scanning the body with a Wood lamp may reveal remnants of dried semen, which fluoresces under ultraviolet light.

Sperm Motility. Aspirate with an eye-dropper material from the posterior fornix of the vagina and place a drop on a slide, cover with a coverslip, and examine under high dry power of the microscope for motile spermatozoa. Record approximate percentage of motile, in relationship to all, sperm seen. Motile sperm may persist in the vagina from 3–24 hours after intercourse. The absence of sperm may be due to the fact that approximately 10% of males are spontaneously oligospermic or aspermic, and the number undergoing vasectomy is rapidly increasing.

Saline Wash and Dry Specimens for Spermatozoa. Areas such as the anus, labia, mouth, and vagina should be swabbed with an applicator and the material smeared onto two slides. The swab itself should then be placed in a tube with 1 cc of isotonic saline, saved, and labeled as to source. Nonmotile sperm have been found in the vagina for up to 17 days.

Acid Phosphatase. This test is generally done if sperm are not seen on direct smear from the vagina, or if there is a suspicious area in the mouth, and routinely from the anus if there is a history or physical findings suggestive of penetration. A cotton-tipped applicator is saturated with the body fluid in any of these locations and then placed in a tube with 1 cc of isotonic saline, covered, labeled, and frozen. Because acid phosphatase is a component of seminal fluid and not normally found in the vagina, mouth, or anus, its presence suggests recent coitus.

Stool Guaiac. This test should be done if there is a history or physical evidence of rectal penetration.

Dipstick of Urine for Occult Blood. This test should be done if there is evidence of traumatic bladder injury and routinely in cases involving children.

VDRL. Because it takes approximately 6 weeks for this test to become positive after exposure, this may be done to serve as a baseline rather than for legal purposes.

Pregnancy Test. Although not required for legal purposes, this test is useful as a baseline in sexually active adolescents to determine if they may have become pregnant prior to the rape. A pregnancy test is mandatory prior to administration of any "morning after" hormone preparation. Either ethinyl estradiol, 5 mg bid for 5 days, or Ovral, two tablets initially and two taken 12 hours later, is effective in preventing pregnancy if administered within 72 hours of unprotected intercourse.

Gonococcal and Chlamydial Cultures. These cultures are useful for treatment rather than for legal purposes.

HIV. Although cases of transmission of HIV to child victims of sexual assault have been reported, it has not *as yet* been recommended that rape victims be followed and tested for it. Judgment should be used in deciding whether patients should be so tested.

INITIAL MANAGEMENT OF THE ADOLESCENT RAPE VICTIM

1. Assess need for emergency care. If not necessary:
2. Reassure patient that he or she is safe and will not suffer any physical sequelae of the ordeal.
3. Listen empathetically.
4. Involve patient in decision making, recognizing that the ability to do this may be temporarily impaired. Therefore if the patient indicates that he or she does not plan to press charges, encourage permission to collect necessary evidence in the event that there is a later change of mind.
5. Get the patient's permission to perform a physical examination, especially a pelvic and/or rectal examination (the antithesis of the rape experience).
6. Prepare the patient for possible emotional sequelae and suggestions for coping with them, including follow-up counseling. It is common for families of children and adolescent victims of rape to impose a cloak of silence, thinking it will help the youngster to forget about what happened. The patient should emphathetically be encouraged to seek followup care.

THE RAPE TRAUMA SYNDROME[8]

Acute Phase

Impact Reactions. These range from the "expressed style" (expressions of fear, anxiety, anger with crying, smiling, and restlessness) to the "controlled style" (feelings are masked or hidden by a calm exterior).

Somatic Reactions. During the first few weeks after the rape, there may be evidence of actual physical trauma, skeletal muscle tension, gastrointestinal irritability and nausea, and genitourinary symptoms, particularly related to the orifice invaded during the rape.

Emotional Reactions. Fear of physical injury or death are most common, with feelings of guilt more common than anger.

Long-term Reorganization Phase

Motor Activity. Whereas adult rape victims often change their place of residence, adolescents typically desire to change their school, even if the rape did not occur in conjunction with school activity.

Nightmares. These may be a reenactment of the rape or often have a theme of "loss of control."

Phobias. Fear of being alone is common, as is fear of crowds. Sexual fears are also very common.

Evaluation of the Adolescent Suspected of Drug Abuse

Drug and alcohol abuse are all too common among today's adolescents. The physician is often called upon when there is a suspicion of drug abuse. The following components of the evaluation will assist making this determination.

History

The goals of the history are to determine if the adolescent is, in fact, using drugs and, if so, to evaluate the cause and potential seriousness of the behavior, as well as possible medical complications.

Taking a Drug History from an Adolescent Patient

At a time when involuntary drug testing is being emotionally debated, the physician's role in obtaining accurate information about drug use by an adolescent and maintaining the confidentiality of such information is in jeopardy. Establishing a good relationship and credibility as the teenager's advocate is crucial. In our experience, teenagers tend to be honest and give accurate information if asked by someone they trust to maintain confidentiality. Asking them to fill out a questionnaire detailing the type, frequency, and amount of the substance used is the most direct and also an effective method for obtaining the necessary information. Alternatively, the following approaches may be useful:

1. The Medical Model. "I am going to give you a prescription for ____. This medication's effectiveness and toxicity can be seriously influenced by the presence of other substances in the blood. Therefore, it is important that you tell me if you have used any pot, alcohol, cigarettes, or drugs within

TABLE 39. Interactions Between Alcohol and Prescription Drugs

Additive	Cross-tolerant	Antagonistic
Acetaminophen	Anticoagulants (chronic intoxication)	Caffeine
Antihypertensives	Digoxin/digitoxin	Cephalosporins
Anticoagulants (acute intoxication)	Ether	Chloramphenacol
Antihistamines	Fluorinated anesthetics	Griseofulvin
Barbiturates	Imipramine	Ketoconazole
Benzodiazepines	Propranolol	Phenformin
Chloral hydrate	Tetracyclines	
Lithium		
Nonsteroidal anti-inflammatory drugs		
Oral contraceptives		
Phenothiazines		
Propoxyphene		
Salicylates		

From Litt IF: Health problems of adolescents. In Behrman RE, Vaughan VC III (eds): Nelson Textbook of Pediatrics. Philadelphia, W.B. Saunders Co., 1987, with permission.

the past month. How about before that? Have you ever tried any of these or other substances?" In conjunction with the medical model, Table 39 lists drug interactions with alcohol and Table 40, with tobacco. The effect of tobacco on laboratory tests is listed in Table 41.

2. The "My friend has a problem" Approach. "It's said that there is a lot of pressure on kids in your school to try drugs. What has been the experience of your friends with such pressures? Have you actually tried any pot, cigarettes, alcohol, or drugs?"

3. The Problem-solving Approach. "What would you do if the friend who drove you to a party became intoxicated from pot or alcohol once you got there? Do you know anyone who has actually had such an experience? Have you?"

4. The Habit Model. "Are there any habits you have thought about wanting to break?"

5. Family Drug or Alcohol Problems. Referring a teenager to ALATEEN, a program for family members of those who have drug or alcohol problems, can help the teenager to learn how to cope with that person, but also may help the adolescent who has or is at risk for developing a similar problem.

EVALUATION OF THE SERIOUSNESS OF DRUG USE (Table 42)

As it is currently normative for most adolescents to experiment with a drug or substance at least once during the high school years, it is important

TABLE 40. Tobacco Interactions with Other Drugs

Acetaminophen	Decreased acetaminophen effect (increased metabolism)	Monitor efficacy
Antidepressants, tricyclic	Decreased antidepressant effect (increased metabolism)	Monitor antidepressant concentration; reported with imipramine, but might occur with other tricyclics
	Possible toxicity with nortriptyline (possibly displacement from binding)	Monitor nortriptyline concentration and maintain at minimal effective dosage; total concentration may be in the therapeutic range, but free concentration elevated
Beta-adrenergic blockers	Decreased propranolol effect (increased metabolism)	Avoid concurrent use; not known whether interaction occurs with other beta-adrenergic blockers
Estrogens	Possible decreased estrogen effect (increased metabolism)	Avoid concurrent use
Insulin	Decreased insulin effect (decreased absorption from injection site)	Avoid concurrent use
Mexiletine	Possible decreased mexiletine effect (increased metabolism)	Monitor mexiletine concentration
Phenylbutazone	Possible decreased phenyl-butazone effect (increased metabolism)	Monitor clinical status
Theophyllines	Decreased theophylline effect (increased metabolism) (also true for smokeless tobacco)	Monitor theophylline concentration

From The Medical Letter Handbook of Adverse Drug Interactions, 1989, p 52, with permission.

for the physician to be able to determine which adolescents are at risk to themselves or others as a result of such behavior. The following factors may be helpful in making such determinations, although the judgment about seriousness should not be made on the basis of any one alone:

Age. The younger the patient who experiments with drugs, the potentially more serious it is. It is useful to have some information about the age of onset of use of various substances for comparative purposes. The median age of onset for cigarette smoking is 11 years; for marijuana use, 13 years; for alcohol use, 14 years; and for cocaine, over the age of 24 years. Onset of use at times earlier than these norms should be regarded as more serious than when they occur at the average age, in terms of being

TABLE 41. Effects of Smoking on Laboratory Tests

Albumin ↓
Carboxyhemoglobin ↑
Carcinoembryonic antigen (CEA) ↑
Cholesterol? ↑
Creatinine ↓
Free fatty acids ↑
Globulin ↓ (women)
Hematocrit ↑
Hemoglobin ↑
Leukocytes ↑
Lymphocytes ↑
Mean cell volume ↑
Nitroblue tetrazolium test (false positive)
Platelet aggregation ↑
Red blood cells ↑
Serum glucose (1 hour post challenge) ↑
Triglycerides ? ↑
Uric acid ↓ (men)
Vitamin C ↓

symptomatic of underlying psychopathology. That is not to say that use at or later than the average time is to be ignored.

Sex. Although use of drugs and alcohol has been increasing among female adolescents recently, it is still more frequent among males. The only exceptions relate to cigarette smoking, and use of diet pills (prescribed and over-the-counter) and psychotropic prescription drugs, all of which are currently more common among female than male adolescents. As with the age criterion above, patterns that differ from the norm may be symptomatic of psychopathology.

Family History of Drug Abuse. Use of drugs by a teenager with a family history of drug abuse is generally considered to be a more serious event in terms of possibly predicting chronic use or addiction and biologic predisposition to associated problems such as depression and bulimia.

Setting of Drug Use. Drug use by the adolescent when he or she is alone is a more serious phenomenon than when this behavior takes place in a group setting.

Affect Prior to Use of Drugs. The adolescent who uses a drug to help to cope with feelings of depression and despair needs psychiatric help, regardless of other factors. Use of drugs at a time when the teenager is happy is of less concern (in and of itself) as a symptom of depression.

School Performance. A teenager who is able to maintain good grades and school attendance is obviously at lower risk from drug experimentation than is one with falling grades and increasing school absenteeism. It is

TABLE 42. Seriousness of Drug Abuse*

	0	+1	+2
Age	>15	>15	
Sex	M	F	
Family history of drug abuse			+
Setting of drug abuse	In group		Alone
Affect before drug use	Happy		Sad
School performance	Good/improving	Always poor	Recently poor
Use before driving			X
History of accidents			X
Time of week	Weekend		Weekdays
Time of day		After school	Before school
Type of drug	Marijuana, beer, wine	Hallucinogens, amphetamines	Whiskey, opiates, cocaine, barbiturates

*Score as follows: 0–3, less worrisome; 3–8, serious; and 9–24, very serious.

important that the teenager be asked about this year's grades and absences compared with last year's, not simply the absolute number. A youngster with a decrement in school performance should be referred for counseling, regardless of other factors.

Use of Drugs in Conjunction with Driving. This is a serious risk factor and requires psychiatric intervention if the primary care physician is unable to change the adolescent's behavior through counseling, reality testing, and role playing.

History of Accidents. As with driving, this requires immediate intervention.

Time of Week and of Day of Use of Drugs. Drug use on the weekend in the company of friends is not as worrisome, in terms of being symptomatic of underlying problems, as is its use during the school week, particularly in the mornings. The latter pattern is quite serious and mandates intervention.

Type of Drug Used. All other things being equal, use of opiates, amphetamines, and barbiturates is more serious than is the use of marijuana or beer. Obviously the latter may be used by a seriously depressed individual who needs psychiatric help or one who may place the life of others in jeopardy by driving while intoxicated, so that the type of drug is not the only criterion for assessing potential seriousness of an adolescent's drug behavior.

PHYSICAL EXAMINATION

This discussion relates to the adolescent who is acutely intoxicated or is suffering from an overdose or drug withdrawal.

General Appearance

Much can be learned simply by observing the adolescent. Malnutrition, a common finding in adult drug abusers who divert any money they get to purchase drugs or alcohol instead of food, is rare in the adolescent, whose nutrition is usually provided by family or custodians. If the patient is comatose, the possibility of drug or alcohol overdose is high in the differential diagnosis. The possibility of diabetic coma, a seizure disorder, or head trauma must also be considered. Slurred speech and ataxic gait suggest the possibility of barbiturate or alcohol overdose. The swearing teenager who is drooling or spitting may do so as the result of use of phencyclidine (PCP).

Vital Signs

Pulse Elevated. Consider stimulants (such as amphetamines, cocaine, methylphenidate, or phenmetrazine); hallucinogens (such as LSD, psilocybin, mescaline, PCP, STP, or MDMA); marijuana, hashish, or THC; and anticholinergics (such as scopolamine or jimsonweed). Withdrawal from narcotics and sedatives also causes tachycardia.

Slow. Narcotics (such as heroin, codeine, methadone, propoxyphene, or meperidine); sedatives (such as secobarbital, amobarbital, chlordiazepoxide, diazepam, methaqualone, or alcohol).

Blood Pressure. *Elevated* (same as for elevated pulse).

Depressed (same as for slow pulse). In addition, anticholinergics (such as scopolamine or jimsonweed) may produce hypotension or hypertension, and a patient in shock from any overdose may also manifest hypotension. Marijuana and related substances may produce postural hypotension. Shock may result from overdose of any drug or alcohol or withdrawal from sedatives.

Temperature. *Hypothermia:* narcotics or shock secondary to overdose of alcohol.

Hyperthermia: hallucinogens (such as LSD, PCP, psilocybin, mescaline, STP, MDMA, etc.); stimulants; anticholinergics; withdrawal from sedatives. Fever may result from brain abscesses or endocarditis in intravenous drug users. These patients are also at risk for AIDS, which typically causes fever.

Respiration. *Shallow:* stimulants.

Depressed: narcotics; sedatives/hypnotics/depressants/tranquilizers.

HEENT

Head. Signs of trauma (such as hematoma and/or Battle sign) should be sought in every teenager who is comatose or obtunded or appears intoxicated. Trauma alone may explain the findings or they may be complications of impairment from drug use.

Eyes. *Pupils.* (1) Constricted: narcotics (particularly opiates, phenothiazines, alcohol, and barbiturates); PCP. (2) Dilated: anticholinergics (fixed); glutethimide; stimulants (reactive); hallucinogens (except PCP); shock from any abused substance; withdrawal from narcotics. (3) Midposition: cannabis group (normally reactive); PCP; sedatives/hypnotics/depressants/tranquilizers group (except for glutethimide) (fixed).

Conjunctivae. Injected drugs in the cannabis group.

Optic Discs. Blurred (volatile inhalants).

Miscellaneous. Blank stare (PCP); nystagmus (PCP; sedatives); tonic-blink reflex (withdrawal from sedatives).

Ears. Hyperacusis (stimulants).

Nose. Hyperemia of nasal mucosa, rare perforation of septum (cocaine).

Dry (anticholinergics).

Mouth. Dry (anticholinergics; stimulants).

Bruxism (amphetamines).

Excessive salivation (PCP; muscarine).

Mucosal lesions mostly in the mandibular mucobuccal fold (chewing tobacco or snuff) (Table 43).

Speech: slurred (sedatives, alcohol).

Breath: foul (stimulants).

Cardiovascular

Arrhythmias: anticholinergics; stimulants (especially cocaine); volatile inhalants.

Murmur of tricuspid insufficiency (in a febrile patient): consider endocarditis secondary to use of unsterile needles.

TABLE 43. Mucosal Lesions Caused by Smokeless Tobacco (Chewing Tobacco or Snuff)

Degree 1:	A superficial lesion with a color similar to the surrounding mucosa with a slight wrinkling, perhaps slight granularity, and no obvious thickening of the surface.
Degree 2:	A superficial reddish or whitish lesion with moderate wrinkling and no obvious thickening.
Degree 3:	A red or white lesion with intervening furrows of normal mucosal color, and with obvious thickening and wrinkling of the surface.

From Greer RO Jr, Poulson TC: Oral tissue alterations associated with the use of smokeless tobacco by teenagers. I. Clinical findings. Oral Surg 56:275–284, 1983, with permission.

Thrombophlebitis (usually superficial) may result from intravenous drug abuse.

Respiratory

Pulmonary edema: narcotics; volatile inhalants.

Pneumonia may result from aspiration. *Pneumocystis carinii* pneumonia in an adolescent is diagnostic of immunosuppression, and AIDS is the likely cause in the IV drug user.

Gastrointestinal

Bowel sounds. *Decreased:* anticholinergics; narcotics.
Increased: stimulants or withdrawal from narcotics or anticholinergics.

Hepatomegaly/Tenderness. Hepatitis in an intravenous drug abuser.

Genitourinary

Urinary retention: anticholinergics.

Renal failure: volatile inhalants.

Musculoskeletal

Increased strength/muscular rigidity (PCP).

Skin

Dry: anticholinergics.

Flushed face: anticholinergics (especially jimsonweed): hallucinogens.

Excessive sweating: stimulants.

Pallor: cannabis group.

Needle tracks: in antecubital fossa, between toes, on dorsum of penis or on foot (narcotics, stimulants).

Tattoos: may be sign of membership in drug subculture or attempt to disguise needle tracks.

Subcutaneous fat necrosis and abscesses: in those who inject drugs subcutaneously.

Pustular acne: may result from amphetamine, LSD or barbiturate use, but is often difficult to differentiate from that commonly found during puberty in the non–drug-using adolescent.

"Gooseflesh": withdrawal from opiates.

Kaposi sarcoma: AIDS in IV drug abusers.

Lymphatic

Lymphadenopathy from bacterial infections or AIDS in intravenous drug abusers.

Neurologic

Convulsions: with overdose of stimulants; propoxyphene; meperidine; methaqualone; anticholinergics; volatile inhalants; or withdrawal from barbiturates, tranquilizers, or glutethimide.

Deep tendon reflexes. *Increased:* anticholinergics; stimulants; hallucinogens (especially PCP). *Depressed:* sedatives; narcotics.

Dysarthria: sedatives, alcohol.

Nystagmus: see eyes, above.

Ataxia: hallucinogens; cannabis group; sedatives.

Tremor: stimulants; withdrawal from narcotics; sedatives.

Peripheral neuropathy: May result from accidental injection into a nerve; toxic effect of chronic toluene abuse.

Hyperactivity: hallucinogens; stimulants.

Parkinsonism: MPTP (N-methyl-4-phenyl-1,2,3,6–tetrahydropyridine)—a street-drug contaminant.

Mental Status Examination

Disorientation: anticholinergics, sedatives; hallucinogens; cannabis group.

Paranoia: hallucinogens; stimulants.

Hallucinations (visual): hallucinogens; cannabis group; anticholinergics (may be auditory as well): stimulants; volatile inhalants.

Body-image alterations: anticholinergics.

Amnesia: hallucinogens; anticholinergics.

Stereotypy: stimulants.

Affect: inappropriate: hallucinogens.

Depersonalization: hallucinogens.

Euphoria: Cannabis group; narcotics; volatile inhalants (transient).

Psychosis: hallucinogens; amphetamines; some volatile inhalants.

Depression: sedatives; stimulant withdrawal.

Evaluation of the Depressed Adolescent

SUICIDE

Suicide is currently the third leading cause of death in 15- to 19-year-olds. Suicide is attempted more often by female teenagers, whereas male adolescents outnumber females in completed suicides. At highest risk are chronically ill adolescents, those with poor self-image, serious students following a failed examination, native American Indians, Eskimos, and Asian-American youth.

Methods

Ingestion of medication is the suicide method most often used by teenagers. This may be the patient's own medication or that of a parent with whom there has been conflict. Currently, the drug most often used in suicide attempts in this country is a tricyclic antidepressant. Table 44 lists drugs commonly used in suicide attempts by adolescents and their toxic levels. Physicians are advised to consider prescribing medication in unit-dose form whenever there is a concern that the patient or a family member may be at risk for suicide.

Seriousness of Intent

Violent methods, such as hanging, shooting, or wrist-slashing, are more often used by males and/or teenagers most intent on killing themselves. It is, however, difficult to assess the seriousness of the suicide intent by the potency of the method. For example, an adolescent who ingests a nontoxic medication (such as antibiotic) may be as serious about committing suicide as is one who consumes a toxic substance. Medical lethality has been found to

TABLE 44. Toxic Levels of Drugs Used in Suicide Attempts by Adolescents

Drug	Source of Specimen	Reference Range	Reference Range (IU)
Acetaminophen	Serum, plasma (heparin, EDTA)	>200 μg/ml	>1300 μmol/L
Amphetamine	Serum, plasma (heparin, EDTA)	>200 ng/ml	>1500 nmol/L
Carbamazepine	Serum, plasma (heparin, EDTA)	>15 μg/ml	>63 μmol/L
Carbon monoxide	Whole blood (EDTA)	>50%	HbCO fraction: >0.5
Diazepam	Serum plasma (heparin, EDTA)	>5000 ng/ml	>17,500 nmol/L
Ethanol	Whole blood (oxylate), serum	50–100 mg/dl Depression of CNS >100 mg/dl	11–22 nmol/L >22 nmol/L
Ethosuximide	Serum, plasma (heparin, EDTA)	>150 μg/ml	>1060 μmol/L
Iron	Serum	>1800 μg/dl	>322.2 μmol/L
Lithium	Serum, plasma (heparin, EDTA)	>2 mmol/L	>2 mmol/L
Phenacetin	Plasma (EDTA)	50–250 μg/ml	280–1400 μmol/L
Phenobarbital	Serum, plasma (heparin, EDTA)	Slowness, ataxia, nystagmus = 35–80 μg/ml Coma with reflexes = 65–117 μg/ml Coma without reflexes >100 μg/ml	150–345 μmol/L 280–504 μmol/L
Phenytoin	Serum, plasma (heparin, EDTA)	>20 μg/ml	>80 μmol/L
Primidone	Serum, plasma (heparin, EDTA)	>15 μg/ml	>69 μmol/L
Salicylates	Serum, plasma (heparin, EDTA)	>30 mg/dl	>2.2 mmol/L
Theophylline	Serum, plasma (heparin, EDTA)	>20 μg/ml	>110 μmol/L
Valproic acid	Serum, plasma (heparin, EDTA)	>100 μg/ml	>700 μmol/L

correlate poorly with the seriousness of intent. A more accurate picture of intent is gained by inquiring of the patient about his or her expectation of lethality (for example, "Did you expect to die as a result of taking these pills?")

In assessing seriousness of suicide attempt, other factors should be considered, including the extent of premeditation and the likelihood of rescue. The adolescent who impulsively grabs a bottle from the medicine cabinet in full view or earshot of his family is generally less serious about committing suicide than is the one who has secretly planned the act, especially if the plan precluded the possibility of rescue. A suicide note implies premeditation and is therefore considered a sign of seriousness of intent. Because numerous studies have shown that most completed suicides occur in people who have made earlier attempts, any suicide attempt or gesture by an adolescent should be treated as serious and as a desperate attempt at resolution of conflict. Attention merely to the surgical or pharmacologic sequelae of the attempt is inadequate to address these needs. Hospitalization of the adolescent is, on the other hand, an effective means of providing a secure setting, of impressing parents of the need to address the underlying problems, and of facilitating the psychosocial assessment, which must provide the data base for appropriate referral and therapy. A skilled psychiatrist should be consulted for every teenager who makes a suicide attempt or gesture.

DEPRESSION

Given the fact that mood swings from the depth of depression to the heights of elation are common during adolescence, it is often difficult to decide which sad-looking adolescent is at risk for true depression and even suicide. The distinguishing factor is the persistence of the depressed mood, the absence of corresponding periods of elation, an inability to function, and the expression of "hopelessness and helplessness." Persistence is defined as a mood that lasts for at least 3 consecutive hours for three or more periods each week.[55]

Symptoms of Depression

Symptoms of depression in the adolescent often include falling (not necessarily "failing") school grades, an increase in school absenteeism or truancy, use of alcohol or drugs, accident-proneness, and pervasive boredom. The opposite mood—persistent euphoria—may be indicative of "masked depression" when coupled with acting-out behavior, such as sexual promiscuity. Vegetative signs, typical of depression in adults, such as disturbances of eating and sleeping, may or may not be found in depressed adolescents. When insomnia does occur in a depressed adolescent, it is typically initial insomnia and difficulty in falling asleep, sometimes to the extent of sleeping all day and remaining awake at night without ever feeling rested. A family history of depression should increase concern, particularly if that history includes a suicide attempt or, especially, a completed suicide.

Interviewing the Depressed Adolescent

In evaluating the adolescent in whom depression is suspected, it is useful to establish whether he or she has plans for the future. The youngster who indicates that he or she has none, or who responds by saying that he or she "won't be here much longer," is obviously a suicide risk. Inquiring whether the patient desires to change anything in his or her life is also an effective way of approaching this subject. If an affirmative answer is elicited, followup questioning should focus on what steps have been taken to make the desired changes. When the patient appears to be depressed, the physician should not hesitate to ask if he or she has ever felt so sad that death was considered a preferable alternative to living. If answered in the affirmative, the existence of a plan for self-destruction should be established. Any patient with a suicide plan must be immediately evaluated by a psychiatrist. Such a line of questioning will not precipitate an attempt, and the patient is often relieved to have an opportunity to discuss concerns with an obviously caring physician. Conversely, the adolescent who suddenly appears cheerful after a period of depression should not be released from care, as such a change may signal a decision to resolve sadness by suicide, rather than be a sign of improvement.

Stages of Depression

Mattsson[36] has described five increasingly pathologic stages or presentations of depression in the adolescent:

1. **Depressive Mood Swings.** These are considered to be normal.

2. **Acute Depressive Reactions.** Following the death or separation from a loved one, depression is a natural experience. In the adolescent, mourning may be the pervasive mood for weeks or months, after which there is gradual movement toward restoration of normal functioning. Close observation and communication with the primary care physician constitute the appropriate management, unless thoughts of suicide or acting-out behavior occurs.

3. **Neurotic Depressive Disorders.** If there is not resolution of the grief reaction following the loss of a loved one, the adolescent may experience feelings of hopelessness and helplessness, self-incrimination and guilt in relationship to the lost individual, difficulty concentrating, withdrawal from school and social contacts, insomnia, anorexia, and decreased

activity. Desire to join the deceased person is often experienced, but is revealed only in response to sensitive inquiry. A psychiatrist is the only professional qualified to manage such a patient.

4. Masked Depression. The adolescent with masked depression responds to feelings of despair by somatization and/or denial. Acting-out behavior, including running away from home, truancy from school, accident-proneness and/or substance abuse, is a common manifestation of this form of depression. Similarly, appearance of headaches, abdominal pain, or other somatic complaints may be symptomatic of masked depression. Such a patient is a candidate for psychiatric therapy.

5. Psychotic Depressive Disorders. The adolescent who, in addition to the above symptoms, manifests impairment of reality testing, distortion of thought, and delusions of guilt, may be suffering from this form of depression. Psychiatric treatment is necessary for such a patient.

Evaluation for Sports Participation

The objectives of the pre-sports participation evaluation during adolescence are threefold:

1. To assess the potential impact of such participation on a known medical problem.
2. To detect any undiagnosed medical condition that may become manifest during athletic activity. If one is detected that is believed to be a contraindication to participating in a particular sport, to channel the adolescent toward another which is compatible with the medical condition.
3. To prevent injury or physiologic dysfunction from planned sports participation.

DISQUALIFYING CONDITIONS FOR SPORTS PARTICIPATION

A list of disqualifying conditions for various types of sports is found in Table 45. For example, it is generally recommended that a teenager with only one of paired vital organs be kept from participating in collision or contact sports in order to prevent injury to the remaining organ.

Hypertension presents a different sort of risk and the guidelines are more flexible. The teenager with moderate hypertension should be prohibited from participating in activities that may increase blood pressure, such as isometric sports (for example, wrestling and weight lifting). Those with mild hypertension might be encouraged to participate in strenuous aerobic exercise, which has been shown to improve cardiovascular fitness and actually lower blood pressure and pulse in studies of adults. The presence of labile hypertension (unsustained blood pressure readings in excess of two standard deviations above the mean for age) is not a contraindication for participation in any athletic activity. If there is any doubt about a given

TABLE 45. Disqualifying Conditions for Sports Participation

Conditions	Collision*	Contact†	Noncontact‡	Other§
General				
Acute infections:				
Respiratory, genitourinary, infectious mononucleosis, hepatitis, active rheumatic fever, active tuberculosis	X	X	X	X
Obvious physical immaturity in comparison with other competitors	X	X		
Hemorrhagic disease:				
Hemophilia, purpura, and other serious bleeding tendencies	X	X	X	
Diabetes, inadequately controlled	X	X	X	X
Diabetes, controlled	††	††	††	††
Jaundice	X	X	X	X
Eyes				
Absence or loss of function of one eye	X	X		
Respiratory				
Tuberculosis (active or symptomatic)	X	X	X	X
Severe pulmonary insufficiency	X	X	X	X
Cardiovascular				
Mitral stenosis, aortic stenosis, aortic insufficiency, coarctation of aorta, cyanotic heart disease, recent carditis of any etiology	X	X	X	X
Hypertension on organic basis	X	X	X	X
Previous heart surgery for congenital or acquired heart disease	‖	‖	‖	‖
Liver, enlarged	X	X		
Skin				
Boils, impetigo, and herpes simplex gladiatorum	X	X		

Reprinted from Sports Medicine: Health Care for Young Athletes, copyright 1983, American Academy of Pediatrics, with permission.

*Football, rugby, hockey, lacrosse, and so forth.

†Baseball, soccer, basketball, wrestling, and so forth.

‡Cross country, track, tennis, crew, swimming, and so forth.

§Bowling, golf, archery, field events, and so forth.

††No exclusions.

‖Each patient should be judged on an individual basis in conjunction with his or her cardiologist and surgeon.

Table continued on opposite page.

teenager, a maximum stress test should be performed in order to assess blood pressure and EKG response to high-intensity exercise in a safe environment. This is appropriate, for example, with a patient with a known cardiovascular problem such as a cardiomyopathy, mitral valve prolapse, or PVCs that will not disappear after low-grade exercise. The presence of any EKG changes or clinical symptoms at rest suggestive of cardiac insufficiency

TABLE 45. Disqualifying Conditions for Sports Participation *(Continued)*

Conditions	Collision*	Contact†	Noncontact‡	Other§
Spleen, enlarged	X	X		
Hernia				
Inguinal or femoral hernia	X	X	X	
Musculoskeletal				
Symptomatic abnormalities or inflammations	X	X	X	X
Functional inadequacy of the musculoskeletal system, congenital or acquired, imcompatible with the contact or skill demands of the sport	X	X	X	
Neurologic				
History or symptoms of previous serious head trauma or repeated concussions	X			
Controlled convulsive disorder	¶	¶	¶	¶
Convulsive disorder not moderately well controlled by medication	X			
Previous surgery on head	X	X		
Renal				
Absence of one kidney	X	X		
Renal disease	X	X	X	X
Genitalia				
Absence of one testicle	**	**	**	**
Undescended testicle	**	**	**	**

¶Each patient should be judged on an individual basis. All things being equal, it is probably better to encourage a young boy or girl to participate in a noncontact sport rather than a contact sport. However, if a patient has a desire to play a contact sport and this is deemed a major ameliorating factor in his or her adjustment to school, associates, and the seizure disorder, serious consideration should be given to letting him or her participate if the seizures are moderately well controlled or the patient is under good medical management.

**The Committee approves the concept of contact sports participation for youths with only one testicle or with an undescended testicle(s), except in specific instances such as an inguinal canal undescended testicle(s), following appropriate medical evaluation to rule out unusual injury risk. However, the athlete, parents, and school authorities should be fully informed that participation in contact sports for youths with only one testicle carries a slight injury risk to the remaining healthy testicle. Fertility may be adversely affected following an injury, but the chances of an injury to a descended testicle are rare, and the injury risk can be further substantially minimized with an athletic supporter and protective device.

should preclude the performance of an exercise stress test and any sports activity.

Detection of asymptomatic conditions known to have caused sudden death during athletic participation among teenagers is the major challenge to the examining primary care physician (Table 46). In addition to a careful physical examination (for murmurs, pulses, anomalies), a family history of early sudden death should be sought. The patient should be asked if he or

TABLE 46. Conditions That Cause Sudden Death in Young Athletes

Hypertrophic obstructive cardiomyopathy
Idiopathic concentric left ventricular hypertrophy
Atherosclerosis
Aberrant origin of the left coronary artery
Hypoplastic coronary arteries
Ruptured aorta

From Smith N, Ogilvie B, Haskell W, et al: Handbook for the Young Athlete. Palo Alto, CA, Bull Publishing Co., 1978, with permission.

she has ever felt faint or actually fainted during exercise. If the response is affirmative, an arrhythmia or an aberrant left coronary artery may be present. Syncope in the post-exercise period, a far more common event, may result from hyperventilation during exercise, and is benign. Chest tightness or shortness of breath following exercise may suggest exercise-induced asthma, a condition that may occur in conjunction with more generalized asthma or in isolation. A patient with exercise-induced asthma may be allowed to participate in sports with the aid of a bronchodilator administered by inhaler before strenuous activity is undertaken.

The positive effects of sports participation for adolescents must be considered in risk-benefit analysis. Every effort should be made to find a substitute sport for the contraindicated one. For example, if collision or contact sports are prohibited for the youngster with a single kidney, the possibility of swimming may be suggested. Disabled teenagers are welcomed in "Special Olympics," and graded exercise programs for those with cardiac conditions exist in most cities.

Prevention of medical complications of sports participation in those without preexisting medical problems is another important task for the physician at the time of the preparticipation evaluation. Many sports injuries can be prevented by matching teams on the basis of physical size (sex, Tanner staging) and by providing appropriate equipment and playing surfaces. Monitoring of iron status by the use of hematocrit and ferritin levels at the beginning and throughout the playing season will prevent the problem of iron deficiency anemia.

References

1. American Academy of Pediatrics: Report of the Committee on Infectious Disease. 1988 Red Book, Elk Grove Village, IL, 1988.
2. American Psychiatric Association: Diagnostic and Statistical Manual of Mental Disorders III-R, Washington, DC, 1987.
3. Becker MH, Nathanson CV, Drachman, RH: Mother's health beliefs and children's clinic visits: A retrospective study. J Commun Health 3:125–135, 1977.
4. Behrman RE, Vaughan VC III (eds): Nelson Textbook of Pediatrics, 13th ed. Philadelphia, W.B. Saunders Co., 1987.
5. Brooks-Gunn J: The psychological significance of different pubertal events to young girls. J Early Adolesc 4:315–327, 1984.
6. Bruch H: The Golden Cage. Cambridge, MA, Harvard University Press, 1978.
7. Brunswick AF: Health needs of adolescence: How the adolescent sees them. Am J Public Health 59:1730–1745, 1969.
8. Burgess AW, Holmstrom LL: Rape Trauma Syndrome. Am J Psychiatry 131:981, 1974.
9. Chess S, Thomas A, Cameron M: Sexual attitudes and behavior patterns in a middle-class adolescent population. Am J Orthopsychiatry 46:689–701, 1976.
10. Cohen MI, Litt IF, Schonberg SK, et al: Perspectives on adolescent medicine: concepts and program design. Acta Paediatr Scand [Suppl] 256:9–16, 1975.
11. Cromer B: Compliance with breast self examination instruction in healthy adolescents. J Adolesc Health Care 10:105–109, 1989.
12. Duke PM: Adolescent sexuality. Pediatr Rev 4:44–52, 1982.
13. Epstein HT: Phrenoblysis: Special brain and mind growth periods. I. Human brain and skull development. Dev Psychobio 7:207–216, 1974.
14. Felice M, Grant J, Reynolds B, et al: Follow-up observations of adolescent rape victims. Clin Pediatr 17:311–315, 1978.
15. Flavell JH: Cognitive Development, 2nd ed. Englewood Cliffs, NJ, Prentice Hall, 1985.
16. Greer RO Jr, Poulson TC: Oral tissue alterations associated with the use of smokeless tobacco by teenagers. I. Clinical findings. Oral Surg 56:275–284, 1983.
17. Greulich WW, Dorfman RI, Catchpole HR, et al: Somatic and endocrine studies of pubertal and adolescent boys. Monogr. Soc Res Child Dev 7(3):1942.
18. Gron AM: Prediction of tooth emergence. J Dent Res 41:573–585, 1962.
19. Gross RT, Duke PM: The effect of early versus late physical maturation on adolescent behavior. Pediatr Clin North Am 27:71–77, 1980.
20. Hill JP, Holmbeck GN: Attachment and autonomy during adolescence. Ann Child Dev 3:145–189, 1986.
21. Kaplan KM, Wadden TA: Childhood obesity and self-esteem. J Pediatr 109:367–370, 1986.

22. Keating D: Cognitive processes in adolescence. In Elliott G, Feldman S (eds): At the Threshold: The Developing Adolescent. Boston, Harvard University Press, 1990.
23. Killen JD, Taylor BC, Telch MJ, et al: Depressive symptoms and substance use among adolescent binge eaters and purgers: A defined population study. Am J Public Health 77:1539–1541, 1987.
24. Kinsey AC, Pomeroy WB, Martin CL: Sexual Behavior in the Human Male. Philadelphia, W.B. Saunders Co., 1953.
25. Kolata G: Obese children: A growing problem. Science 232:20–21, 1986.
26. Levine MD: Developmental variations and dysfunctions in the school child. In Levine MD, Carey WB, Crocker AC, Gross RT (eds): Developmental–Behavioral Pediatrics. Philadelphia, W.B. Saunders Co., 1983.
27. Litt IF: Adolescent health as we enter the '80's. In Coates JJ, Peterson AC, Perry C (eds): Promoting Adolescent Health: A Dialog on Research and Practice. New York, Academic Press, 1982.
28. Litt IF: Adolescent health care. In Green M, Haggerty RJ (eds): Ambulatory Pediatrics III. Philadelphia, W.B. Saunders Co., 1984, pp 80–103.
29. Litt IF: Compliance with pediatric medication regimens. In Yaffe SJ (ed): Pediatric Pharmacology, Therapeutic Principles in Practice, 2nd ed. Orlando, FL, Grune and Stratton, in press.
30. Litt IF: Menstrual problems during adolescence. Pediatr Rev 4:203, 1983.
31. Litt IF, Cuskey, WR: Satisfaction with health care: A predictor of adolescents' appointment keeping. J Adolesc Health Care 5:196–200, 1984.
32. Litt IF, Cuskey WR, Rudd S: Identifying the adolescent at risk for contraceptive noncompliance. J Pediatr 96:742–745, 1980.
33. Litt IF, Steinerman PR: Compliance with automotive safety devices among adolescents. J Pediatr 99:484–486, 1981.
34. Macfarlane A, McPherson A, McPherson K, et al: Teenagers and their health. Arch Dis Child 62:1125–1129, 1987.
35. Marino DD, King JC: Nutritional concerns during adolescence. Pediatr Clin North Am 27:125–139, 1980.
36. Mattsson A: Adolescent depression and suicide. In Friedman SB, Hoekelman RA (eds): Behavioral Pediatrics. New York, McGraw-Hill, 1980.
37. Mechanic D: Adolescent health and illness behavior: Review of the literature and a new hypothesis for the study of stress. J Human Stress 9:4–13, 1983.
38. Mellin L, et al: Evidence of reactive obesity in adolescent females. Presented at Annual Meeting, Society for Adolescent Medicine, New York, 1982.
39. Mendoza F, Litt IF, Moss N, et al: Ethnic differences in patient-provider interactions in prenatal care. Pediatr Res 21: 176A, 1987.
40. Millstein, SG: The potential of school-linked centers to promote adolescent health and development. Carnegie Council on Adolescent Development, 1988.
41. Millstein SG, Irwin CZ: Concepts of health and illness: Different constructs or variations on a theme? Health Psychol 6:515–524, 1987.
42. Nielson CT, Skakkebaek NE, Richardson DW, et al: Onset of the release of spermatozoa (spermarche) in boys in relation to age, testicular growth, pubic hair, and height. J Clin Endocrinol 62:532–535, 1986.
43. Nydick M. Bustos J, Dale JH, et al: Gynecomastia in adolescent boys. JAMA 178:449–454, 1961.
44. Offer D: The Psychological World of the Teenager. New York, Basic Books, 1973.
45. Ogden JA: Skeletal Injury in the Child. Philadelphia, Lea and Febiger, 1982, pp 56–57.
46. Overby KJ, Lo B, Litt IF: Knowledge and concerns about AIDS and their relationship to behavior among adolescents with hemophilia. Pediatrics 83:204–210, 1989.

47. Palla BG, Litt IF: Medical complications of eating disorders in adolescents. Pediatrics 81:613–623, 1988.
48. Pantell RH, Goodman BW: Adolescent chest pain: A prospective study. Pediatrics 71: 881–887, 1983.
49. Parcel GS, Nader PR, Meyer MO: Adolescent health concerns, problems, and patterns of utilization in a triethnic urban population. Pediatrics 60: 157–164, 1977.
50. Peck EB, Uldrich ND: Children and weight: A changing perspective. Berkeley, CA, Nutrition Committee Association, 1985.
51. Piaget J (The work of Piaget has been revised and summarized by Flavell JH: The Developmental Psychology of Jean Piaget, Princeton NJ, van Nostrand, 1963; and by Rosen H: Piagetian Dimensions of Clinical Relevance. New York, Columbia University Press, 1985.)
52. Piers EV, Harris D: Age and other correlates of self-concept in children. Educ Psychol 55:91–95, 1964.
53. Pillsbury DM, Shelley WB, Kligman AM: A Manual of Cutaneous Medicine, Philadelphia, W.B. Saunders Co., 1961.
54. Piver C, Litt IF: Rubella screening in adolescent females. Presented at meeting of Western Society for Pediatric Research, Carmel, CA, February 3, 1989.
55. Puig-Antich J. Rabinovich H: Major child and adolescent psychiatric disorders. In Levine MD, Carey WB, Crocker AC, Gross RT (eds): Developmental–Behavioral Pediatrics, W.B. Saunders Co., Philadelphia, 1983, pp 865–890.
56. Rowland TW, Black SA, Kelleher JK: Iron deficiency in adolescent endurance athletes. J Adolesc Health Care 8:322–326, 1987.
57. Schildkrout SM, Shenker R: Human Figure Drawings in Adolescence. New York, Brunner/Mazel, Inc., 1972.
58. Schofield BS: The Sexual Behavior of Young People. Boston, Little, Brown and Co., 1965.
59. Smith N, Ogilvie B, Haskell W, et al: Handbook for the Young Athlete. Palo Alto, CA, Bull Publishing Company, 1978.
60. Sorensen R: Adolescent Sexuality in Contemporary America. New York, World Press Co., 1973.
61. Steinberg L: Reciprocal relation between parent-child distance and pubertal maturation. Dev Psychol 24:1–7, 1988.
62. Strober M: Subclassification of anorexia nervosa: psychologic and biologic correlates. In: Understanding Anorexia Nervosa and Bulimia. Columbus, OH, Ross Laboratories, 1983.
63. Tanner JM: Growth at Adolescence, 2nd Ed. Oxford, Blackwell Scientific Publishers, 1962.
64. Tanner JM: Fetus into Man: Physical Growth from Conception to Maturity. Cambridge, MA, Harvard University Press, 1978.
65. Theander S: Anorexia nervosa: A psychiatric investigation of 94 female cases. Acta Psychiatry Scand [Suppl.] 214:1–194, 1970.

Appendices

APPENDIX 1

Stanford Youth Clinic
Medical History Form

Parent to complete Part I

I. **Past Medical History**

A. **Birth:**

1. Medications during pregnancy?
   yes _____ name of medication(s) ____________________
   no _____
2. Was pregnancy full term (9 mos.)? yes _____ no _____
3. Did patient stay in hospital after mother went home?
   yes _____ why? ____________________
   no _____

B. **Past Illnesses:**
(Please provide dates)
Rheumatic fever ____________ Chickenpox ____________
Tuberculosis ____________ Measles ____________
Hepatitis ____________ Mumps ____________
V.D. (syphilis, gonorrhea, etc.) ____________________
German measles (rubella) ____________________
Other ____________________

C. **Immunizations:**
(Please include dates of last immunizations)
DPT (Diphtheria, Pertussis, Tetanus) ____________________
DT (Diphtheria, Tetanus) ____________________
Polio (by mouth) ____________________
Measles ____________________
Mumps ____________________
German Measles (Rubella) ____________________
Smallpox ____________________
B.C.G. ____________________
T.B. test ____________________
Others ____________________

D. **Hospitalization:**
1. Overnight stay(s) in hospital?
Date ____________ Reason ____________
Date ____________ Reason ____________
2. Surgery?
Date ____________ Reason ____________

E. **Allergies:**

1. Medication (which one(s)) ______

   type of reaction ______

2. Food(s) ______

   type of reaction ______

3. Other ______

   ______

   type of reaction ______

Patient to complete Part II

THE INFORMATION YOU PROVIDE IS CONFIDENTIAL AND FOR THE SOLE USE OF THE STAFF OF THE YOUTH CLINIC WHO WILL NEED IT IN ORDER TO BETTER MEET YOUR HEALTH CARE NEEDS.

II. **Personal Information**

A. **Present medications or drugs** (include vitamins, self-administered drugs, street drugs, etc.)

Name	Dose	How Often	Reason	Prescribed by M.D.?

B. **Diet:**

1. Regular   Yes ____ No ____
2. Special: Type ______
2. For how long ______
2. For what reason ______

C. **Habits:**

1. Any habits you would like to break?

   List: ______

   ______

2. Do you drink alcohol-containing beverages?

   Yes ____ No ____

   If yes, how much each day? ______ or each week ______

   What type? Beer; Wine; Whiskey; Other ______
   (circle all that apply)

   How old were you when you first began to drink? ______

Do you drink when you are: happy; sad; alone;
(circle all that apply) worried; in a group;
other ______________________

3. Do you smoke? Yes _____ No _____
If yes, how many each day? ______________________
What type cigarettes; joints; other ______________________
(circle)

How old were you when you first began to smoke? __________
Do you want to quit? ______________________

4. Do you use smokeless tobacco (e.g., snuff, chew)?
Yes _____ No _____
If yes, for how long? ______________________

D. Below are listed a number of common problems reported to us by other teenagers. Answer each question by checking either yes, no, or n/a (does not apply), so that we may be in a better position to help you.

		Yes	No	N/A
1.	Trouble falling asleep	_____	_____	_____
2.	Awakening during the night	_____	_____	_____
3.	Being very tired during the day . . .	_____	_____	_____
4.	Occasionally wetting the bed	_____	_____	_____
5.	Pain with menstrual period	_____	_____	_____
6.	Bothered by headaches	_____	_____	_____
7.	Bothered by stomach aches	_____	_____	_____
8.	Bothered by dizzy spells	_____	_____	_____
9.	Bothered by leg pains	_____	_____	_____
10.	Worrying about health	_____	_____	_____
11.	Concerned that I am too short . . .	_____	_____	_____
12.	Concerned that I am too tall	_____	_____	_____
13.	Concerned that I am too thin	_____	_____	_____
14.	Concerned that I am too fat	_____	_____	_____
15.	Concerned that my breasts are too small	_____	_____	_____
16.	Concerned that my breasts are too big	_____	_____	_____
17.	Concerned that my penis is too small	_____	_____	_____
18.	Worried that I might become pregnant before I am ready	_____	_____	_____
19.	Worried that I might make someone pregnant	_____	_____	_____
20.	I have questions about my sexual preference	_____	_____	_____

		Yes	No	N/A
21.	Worried that I might not be able to get pregnant or make someone pregnant	_____	_____	_____
22.	Not yet ready for sex, but feel pressured	_____	_____	_____
23.	Worried about AIDS	_____	_____	_____
24.	Worried about my parents' relationship	_____	_____	_____
25.	I would like to change something in my relationship with my parents . .	_____	_____	_____
26.	Do you have a friend you can talk to about anything at all?	_____	_____	_____
27.	Trouble getting to school	_____	_____	_____
28.	Worried about school	_____	_____	_____
29.	Troubled about future plans	_____	_____	_____
30.	Sometimes I'm so sad that I think about dying	_____	_____	_____
31.	Have other personal problems which I would like to discuss with the doctor, but rather not write down	_____	_____	_____

E. **Family History:**

1. Is there anyone in the family whose health worries you?

____

2. List family members:

Name	Age	Living at home?	Any health problems?
Mother			
Father			
Sisters			
Brothers			

F. **When was the last time:**

1. you had a checkup by a doctor? (please include doctor's name)

____

2. you had a checkup by a dentist? _______________
3. you had your vision checked? _______________
4. you had your hearing checked? _______________
5. you had a pelvic/Pap smear? _______________

G. **Safety:**

1. Do you drive a car? Yes _____ No _____
2. Do you:

always use a seat belt?
sometimes use a seat belt? (circle one)
never use a seat belt?

3. Do you ride a:

 motorcycle, bike (circle all that apply)

 If yes, do you:

 always wear a helmet?
 sometimes wear a helmet?
 never wear a helmet?

4. If yes to 1 or 3, do you:

 sometimes drink alcohol before driving? Yes _____ No _____
 sometimes smoke a joint before driving? Yes _____ No _____

APPENDIX 2

The Piers-Harris Children's Self-Concept Scale*

Physical Appearance and Attributes	YES	NO
1. My looks bother me	________	________
2. My friends like my ideas	________	________
3. I have pretty eyes	________	________
4. I am a leader in games and sports	________	________
5. I am popular with girls	________	________

* Subscale from the Piers-Harris Children's Self-Concept Scale, Ellen V. Piers, Ph.D. and Dale B. Harris, Ph.D., 1969, Western Psychological Services, Los Angeles, CA, with permission.

APPENDIX 3

Autonomy Scale

	YES	NOT SURE	NO
1. Do you often find life difficult to cope with?	______	______	______
2. Do you often get the feeling that it's no use trying to get anywhere in life?	______	______	______
3. Do you often feel that you don't have enough control over the direction that your life is taking?	______	______	______
4. Do you find that things are changing so fast today that it's difficult to know what rules to follow?	______	______	______
5. Do you often get the feeling that other people are using you?	______	______	______

APPENDIX 4

Adolescent Compliance Prediction Checklist

	Score
Health Beliefs	
1. Patient believes he/she is susceptible to recurrence (or to disease if prophylactic treatment)	Yes = 1
2. Patient (and/or parent) believes the disease is serious (regardless of actual seriousness)	Yes = 1
3. Patient believes that treatment is efficacious	Yes = 1
4. Agrees with statement: "I try to do exactly what the doctor tells me to do, without question."	Yes = 2
Reality Factors	
1. Actual experience with the disease	
a) Duration	<6 mos = 1
b) Complications of disease	Yes = 1
c) Knowledge of others with the disease	Yes = 1
2. Experience with the medication	
a) Side effects in past	No = 1
b) Sequelae when stopped in past	Yes = 1
c) History of difficulty remembering medications in past	No = 2
3. Relationship to health care provider	
a) Continuous	Yes = 2
b) Satisfied with relationship	Yes = 2
Developmental Factors	
1. Chronological age	>15 = 1
2. Tanner stage	>3 = 1
3. History of responsible autonomous behavior (after-school job; makes and cancels own appointments; assumes responsibility for taking medications, etc.)	Yes = 1
4. Self-image	Positive = 1
5. Depression	No = 1

Expected compliance: Good (13–20)
Questionable (6–12)
Poor (0–5)

APPENDIX 5

Eating Disorder Inventory Scale*

ALWAYS	USUALLY	OFTEN	SOMETIMES	RARELY	NEVER	
___	___	___	___	___	___	1. I eat sweets and carbohydrates without feeling nervous.
___	___	___	___	___	___	2. I think about dieting.
___	___	___	___	___	___	3. I feel extremely guilty about overeating.
___	___	___	___	___	___	4. I am terrified of gaining weight.
___	___	___	___	___	___	5. I exaggerate or magnify the importance of weight.
___	___	___	___	___	___	6. I am preoccupied with the desire to be thinner.
___	___	___	___	___	___	7. If I gain a pound, I worry that I will keep gaining.

*Drive for thinness subscale as taken from the EDI scale. Adapted and reproduced by special permission of Psychological Assessment Resources, Inc., 16204 North Florida Avenue, Lutz, Florida 33549, from The Eating Disorder Inventory, by Garner, Olmstead, Polivy. Copyright 1984 by Psychological Assessment Resources, Inc. Further reproduction is prohibited without prior permission from PAR, Inc.

APPENDIX 6

The Beck Depression Inventory*

On this questionnaire are groups of statements. Please read each group of statements carefully. Then pick out the one statement in each group which best describes the way you have been feeling the past week, including today! Circle the number beside the statement you picked. If several statements in the group seem to apply equally well, circle each one. Be sure to read all the statements in each group before making your choice.

1. 0 I do not feel like a failure
   1 I feel I have failed more than the average person
   2 As I look back on my life, all I can see is a lot of failures
   3 I feel I am a complete failure as a person

2. 0 I don't get more tired than usual
   1 I get tired more easily
   2 I get tired from doing almost anything
   3 I am too tired to do anything

*The sample statements above are drawn from the Beck Depression Inventory, Copyright 1987 by Aaron T. Beck, M.D., Reproduced by permission of the publisher, The Psychological Corporation, 555 Academic Court, San Antonio, Texas 78204-2498. All rights reserved.

APPENDIX 7

Technique of Pelvic Examination in an Adolescent

1. Have the patient placed in lithotomy position after general examination is completed.

2. **Inspection:** of the pubis for Tanner staging, or for pediculosis; of the external genitalia for malformations, lesions, lacerations, bleeding or discharge; and of the vaginal mucosa for evidence of excoriation.

   A foul odor would suggest a foreign body, gonorrhea or trichomonas, whereas an acrid odor would suggest candidosis.

   The hymen is next viewed to determine if it is intact or imperforate. The vagina is examined for bleeding and the urethra inspected for inflammation, caruncle or prolapse. The size of the clitoris is noted.

3. **Digital examination:** A gloved, non-lubricated finger is inserted. The mucosa normally feels rugose. Are there any polyps or masses? Does the cervix point forward or backward? Does it feel soft or firm (like the tip of a nose)? Is there any irregularity, nodularity or tenderness on palpation of the tip of the cervix? Do you feel strings or plastic at the os (when IUD has been placed)?

4. **Bimanual examination:** Place the other hand on the abdomen and gently push down in the midline until you feel downward pressure on cervix. This will allow you to judge the height of the uterine fundus, which normally is below the pelvic brim.

   Next palpate the adnexa. The ovaries should be about the size of walnuts. Don't be alarmed if you cannot feel the ovaries. Is there marked asymmetry in ovarian size or a discrete mass or marked tenderness upon palpation?

   Finally, gently rock the cervix and note the patient's reaction. If there is marked abdominal tenderness on cervical motion in either or both directions this would suggest inflammation or a mass in the tube or ligaments of the uterus.

5. **Speculum examination:** This is done in order to visualize the vaginal vault and cervix, and to facilitate obtaining specimens for a Pap smear and cultures.

Technique of Pelvic Examination *(Continued)*

A disposable plastic speculum is preferable, since it allows visualization of the entire vaginal vault, is more comfortable for the patient and can be connected to its own fiberoptic light source. The speculum may be lubricated, unless cultures and Pap smears are to be taken, in which case lubricant should be avoided.

Introduce the closed speculum with its narrowest diameter perpendicular to the labia (the handle pointing to the thigh) while the index finger of the opposite hand applies pressure posteriorly at the fourchette. Once the speculum is inserted as far posteriorly as it goes with ease, the handle is turned medially, so that it points toward the anus, and the speculum is opened. The cervix is inspected for lacerations, lesions, cyanosis, or discharge from the os.

A sterile swab is inserted into the os and then discarded, after which subsequent swabs may be inserted into the os for cultures.

Pap smears are obtained as follows: the wider end of the spatula is inserted into the cervical os and rotated in order to obtain a sample of endocervical cells. The thinner end is inserted and rotated in such a way as to obtain a specimen from the vaginal fornix.

The specimens are spread on separate slides and *immediately* sprayed with a fixative.

Many physicians perform the speculum examination before the digital and bimanual evaluations. We prefer to do the speculum examination last, since it is the part most feared by adolescents. When the more comfortable maneuver is done first, the patient may relax and become more receptive to later insertion of a speculum.

If a pelvic examination is refused and cultures are necessary, an attempt should be made to insert a swab far into the vagina for culture, or (less satisfactorily) to have the patient do this herself under the physician's guidance.

APPENDIX 8

Laboratory Values Specific for Adolescents

Test	Specimen Source	Age (yr)/Pubertal Stage	Reference Range F	Reference Range M	Reference Range in International Units F	Reference Range in International Units M
Aldosterone	P,S	11–15/	<5–50	ng/dl	<0.14–1.4	nmol/L
					F	M
Alkaline	S	/1			51–108	43–130 IU/L
Phosphatase		/2			49–138	42–204
		/3			26–148	46–240
		/4			16–144	32–228
		/5			13–76	21–228
Albumin	S		3.5–5.0 g/dl		35–50 g/L	
Catecholamines	U,24h	6–15/	20–80 μg/d		20–80 μg/d	
(total free)		>15/	30–100 μg/d		30–100 μg/d	
Cholesterol,	S,P	/1			3.5–6.7	3.1–5.9 mmol/L
total		/2			3.4–6.9	3.0–6.3
		/3	<210 mg/dl		2.9–5.6	2.9–5.2
		/4			3.2–6.6	3.1–5.1
		/5			3.1–6.4	3.0–5.1
Copper	S	12/	80–160 μg/dl		12.56–25.12 μmol/L	
Cortisol (free)	U,24h	Adol.	5–55 μg/dl		14–152 nmol/d	
Creatinine	S,P	/1			42–58	39–63 μmol/L
		/2			36–70	46–73
		/3			39–78	44–80
		/4			44–76	33–90
		/5			48–76	44–90

Continued on next page.

Laboratory Values Specific for Adolescents *(Continued)*

Test	Specimen Source	Age (yr)/Pubertal Stage	Reference Range F	Reference Range M	Reference Range in International Units F	Reference Range in International Units M
Dehydroepi-androsterone (DHEA)	U,24h	10–15/	<0.4 mg/d		<1.4 μmol/d	
Dihydrotes-tosterone (DHT)	S	/1	<10	<10 ng/dl	<0.34	<0.3 nmol/L
		/2	<15	<20	<0.5	<0.7
		/3	<25	<35	<0.86	<1.2
		/4–5	<25	<75	<0.86	<2.6
Estradiol	S,P	/1	0–23	2–8 pg/ml	0–84	7–29 pmol/L
		/2	0–66	11	0–242	40
		/3	0–105	<20	0–385	<73
		/4	20–300	—	73–1101	—
		/5		8–36	—	29–132
	Follicular		10–90		37–330	
	Midcycle		100–500		367–1835	
	Luteal		50–240		184–881	
FSH	S,P	midcycle peak			10–90	
		/1	0.5–8.1	0.5–10.2 mIU/ml		
		/2	0.7–10.0	0.5–10.0		
		/3	0.8–15.0	1.0–18.0		
		/4	1.2–20.0	1.0–20.0		
		/5	1.3–20.0	1.0–30.0		
HDL-Cholesterol	S,P	15–19/	30–70	30–65 mg/dl	.78–1.81	.78–1.68 mmol/L
Hematocrit		/1	34.6–42.1	35.2–41.8%		
		/2	35.7–42.1	36.0–42.8		
		/3	35.2–42.6	37.3–43.5		
		/4	34.9–42.8	38.3–44.8		
		/5	35.9–42.2	39.6–46.4		

17-Hydroxy-progesterone	S	/1	0.2–0.5	0.1–0.3 ng/ml	0.6–1.5	0.3–0.9 nmol/L
		Follicular	0.2–0.8		0.6–2.4	
		Luteal	0.8–3.0		2.4–9.0	
Immunoglobulin A (IgA)	S	12–16/	81–232 mg/dl		810–2320 mg/L	
Immunoglobulin G (IgG)	S	12–16/	700–1550 mg/dl		7–15.5 g/L	
Immunoglobulin M (IgM)	S	12–16/	45–240 mg/dl		450–2400 mg/L	
17-Ketogenic steroids	U,24h	11–14/	<12 mg/d		<42 μmol/d	
		>14/	3–15	5–23	10–52	17–80
17-Ketosteroids, total	U,24h	12–14/	3–10 mg/d		10–35 μmol/d	
		14–16/	5–12 mg/d		17–42 μmol/d	
LH	P	/1	0.2–7.5	0.2–10.3 mIU/ml		
		/2	0.4–11.5	0.5–12.0		
		/3	0.5–15.0	0.5–15.0		
		/4	0.6–34.0	0.6–20.0		
		/5	0.5–80.0	0.5–25.0		
Metanephrine	U,24h	10–15/	0.001–1.87 μg/mg creatinine		0.0006–1.07 mmol/mol creatinine	
		15–18/	0.001–0.67 μg/mg		0.0006–0.38 mmol/mol	
Phosphorus	P	/1			1.1–1.5	1.1–1.5 mmol/L
		/2			1.0–1.6	1.0–1.5
		/3			1.0–1.4	1.2–1.5
		/4			0.9–1.4	1.0–1.5
		/5			0.9–1.3	0.9–1.3
Pregnanetriol	U	<15/	<1.5 mg/d		<4.5 μmol/d	
		>15/	<2.0 mg/d		<5.9 μmol/d	
Progesterone	S		0.11–0.26 ng/ml		0.35–0.83 nmol/L	
		/1	0–0.3		0–1	
		/2	0–0.46		0–1.5	
		/3	0–0.6		0–2	
		/4	.05–13.0		.16–41	
	Follicular		.02–0.9		.06–2.9	
	Luteal		6.0–30.0		19–95	

Laboratory Values Specific for Adolescents *(Continued)*

Test	Specimen Source	Age (yr)/Pubertal Stage	Reference Range		Reference Range in International Units	
			F	*M*	*F*	*M*
Prolactin (hPRL)	S	/1	3.8–13.5	3.6–10.3 mIU/ml		
		/2	3.1–11.7	2.4–18.9		
		/3	3.8–19.2	3.0–15.2		
		/4	4.2–16.8	4.3–18.1		
		/5	5.0–18.0	3.1–15.7		
Protein	CSF	Adol.	15–20 mg/dl		150–200 mg/L	
	U	>13/	<148.4 ug/ml		(<178.1 μg protein/mg creatinine)	
Renin	P	12–15/	<4.2 ng/ml/hr		<4.2 μg/L/hr	
	(EDTA)	15–18/	<4.3 ng/ml/hr		<4.3	
Reverse tri-iodothyronine (rT_3)	S	10–15/	19–88 ng/dl		0.29–1.36 nmol/L	
Riboflavin (Vit. B2)	U	10–15/	200–400 μg/g creatinine		60–120 μmol/ml creatinine	
Somatomedin-C	P	/1	0.8–1.8	0.7–1.1 U/ml		
		/2	0.6–2.6	0.8–2.2		
		/3	2.0–4.2	1.4–2.4		
		/4	2.0–4.2	1.4–2.4		
		/5	2.0–4.2	2.0–3.2		
Testosterone, total	S	/1	2–18	3–110 ng/dl		
		/2	14–65	2–300		
		/3	19–80	27–910		
		/4	20–85	92–840		
		/5	20–85	200–1000		

Thiamine (Vit. B1)	U acidified	13–15/	151–250 μg/g creatinine		64–107 μmol/ml creatinine	
Thyroid-stimulating hormone (RIA)	S	/1	10.5	8.5 uU/ml		
		/2	9.8	8.7		
		/3	7.4	10.8		
		/4	8.3	12.5		
		/5	8.9	15.7		
Thyroxine (RIA)		/1	10.1	10.7 mg/dl		
		/2	10.3	9.4		
		/3	10.2	8.9		
		/4	8.9	8.5		
		/5	10.8	8.4		
Thyroxine-binding globulin (TBG)	S	10–15/	2.1–4.6 mg/dl		21–46 mg/L	
		>15/	1.5–3.4 mg/dl		13–34 mg/L	
Triglycerides	S fasting	12–15/	41–138	36–138 mg/dl	.41–1.38	.36–1.38 g/L
		16–19/	40–128	40–163	.40–1.28	.40–1.63
Triiodo-thyronine, total (t_3-RIA)	S	10–15/	80–120 ng/dl		1.23–3.23 nmol/L	
		>15/	115–190		1.77–2.93	
Urates	P	/1			183–361	121–384 μmol/L
		/2			161–389	123–390
		/3			167–380	165–428
		/4			166–397	224–429
		/5			163–376	218–454
Urine volume	U(24h)	Adol.	700–1400 ml/d		0.700–1.400 L/d	
VMA	U(24h)	Adol.	1–5 mg/d		5–25 μmol/d	

Modified from: (1) Mabry CC. In Behrman RE, Vaughan VC (eds): Nelson Textbook of Pediatrics, 13th ed. Philadelphia, W.B. Saunders, 1987; (2) Copeland K, Brookman RR, Rauh JL: Assessment of Pubertal Development. Ross Laboratories, August 1986; (3) Boineau FG, Lewy JE: Evaluation of hematuria in children and adolescents. Pediatr Rev 11:104, 1989.

Index

Entries in **boldface type** indicate complete chapters.